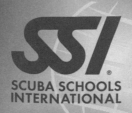

SCUBA SCHOOLS
INTERNATIONAL

DIVER
Stress &
Rescue

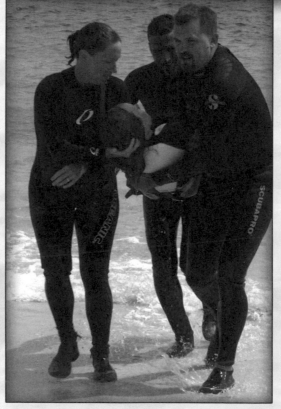

DISCLAIMER:

The information contained in the SSI training materials is intended to give an individual enrolled in a training course a broad perspective of the diving activity. There are many recommendations and suggestions regarding the use of standard and specialized equipment for the activity. Not all of the equipment discussed in the training material can, or will, be used in this activity. The choice of equipment and techniques used in the course is determined by the location of the activity, the environmental conditions and other factors.

A choice of equipment and techniques cannot be made until the dive site is surveyed immediately prior to the dive. Based on the dive site, the decision should be made regarding which equipment and techniques shall be used. The decision belongs to the dive leader and the individual enrolled in the training course.

The intent of all SSI training materials is to give individuals as much information as possible in order for individuals to make their own decisions regarding the diving activity, what equipment should be used and what specific techniques may be needed. The ultimate decision on when and how to dive is for the individual diver to make.

First Edition
　　First Printing, 1/91
　　First Revision, 12/93
　　Second Revision, 11/95
　　Third Revision, 10/00

Second Edition
　　First Printing, 7/05
　　Second Printing 7/07
　　Third Prinitng 9/09

PRINTED IN THE USA!

This manual is printed using Low-VOC ink.

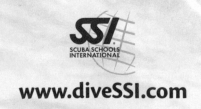

www.diveSSI.com

Contents

Part 1: Stress

Part 2: Rescue

Acknowledgements

Editor in Chief	Doug McNeese
Manager of Development	Suzanne Fletcher
Graphic Designers	Lori Evans, Jennifer Silos,
Cover Photo	SSI Staff
Photographers	SSI Staff Randy Pfizenmaier
Contributing Photographers	Martin Denison, Black Durgeon, Paolo Lilla, Rick Murchison, SSI Australia
Technical Editors	Dr. Art Bachrach, Ph.D.; Daryl Bauer; Paul Caputo; Watson DeVore; Brian Foley, M.Sc.; Dr. Art Hardy, M.D.; Bruce Jameson; Douglas Kelley; Dr. Bert Kobayashi, Ph.D.; Steve Linton; Doug McNeese; David Morgridge; Kirk Mortensen; Frank Palmero; Eric Peterson; Ed Salamone; Dr. Paul Thombs, M.D.

Preface

You will see that each section includes several unique icons to highlight information or add information that relates to the text near it. In some cases, these icons point out information directly associated with the section objectives, while in other cases, the icon indicates a continuing education opportunity. While these icons are designed to help you learn and retain information, they also provide you with an easy reference to important information as you study.

Pearl

"Pearl" the oyster (originally named "Hey!"), is found throughout the text to point out information that we believe is key to a new diver's success. The "pearls of wisdom" that our oyster friend highlights are designed to help you meet section objectives, assist in answering study guide questions and may be used in group discussions with your instructor.

Continuing Education

At Scuba Schools International, we believe that one of the keys to achieving and maintaining success as a diver is taking the "next step" via continuing education. To reinforce that belief, we have put a Continuing Education icon next to topics that correspond to continuing education opportunities available to you through your SSI Dealer. Your SSI Instructor or Dealer will be happy to answer any questions you may have about the continuing education courses listed throughout this manual.

Environment

SSI has always supported and promoted environmental awareness and believes that care for the environment should be a standard part of diver education from start to finish. For these reasons, an environmental icon has been included to highlight important environmental issues as they relate to divers and the underwater world. Topics that you will find the environmental icon next to include the importance of buoyancy control, reef appreciation and conservation, and using your equipment in an environmentally friendly way.

International Use

To meet international English language recommendations, some of the words you come across in this manual may look misspelled. The following is a list of these words in American English and their International counterparts.

American English	International Counterpart
Center	Centre
Meter	Metre
Gray	Grey
Aluminum	Aluminium

Throughout the manual, imperial measurements are listed first followed by the metric conversion. The following conversion units were used to convert the various measurements:

1 ATA (Atmospheres Absolute) = 14.7 psi (pounds per square inch)

1 ATA = 33 fsw (feet of sea water)

1 ATA = 10.33 metres of sea water

1 ATA = 1 bar

1 Metre = 3.28 feet

$C° = (F° - 32) \div 1.8$

1 kg (kilogram) = 2.2 lbs (pounds)

1 km (kilometre) = .621 miles

Note: For greater ease, many of the conversions in this text have been rounded to the nearest whole number, and may not reflect the exact conversion.

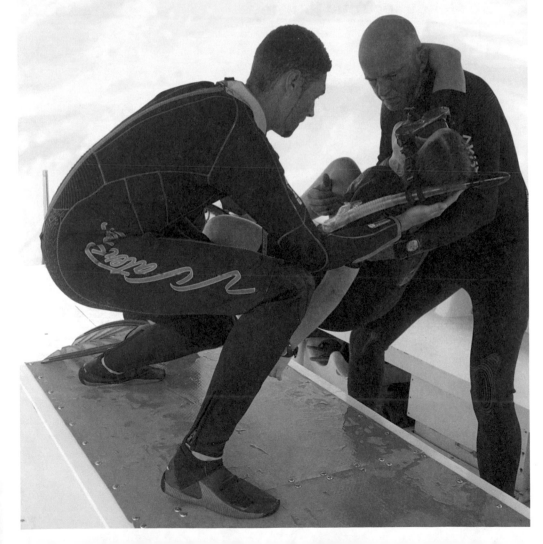

Be Ready
for Your
Journey

SSI.
SCUBA SCHOOLS
INTERNATIONAL

Welcome

Stress is a major contributor to rescue situations and diving accidents. You can improve your diving confidence and enjoyment by learning to recognize, handle and prevent stress related situations.

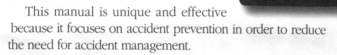

This manual is unique and effective because it focuses on accident prevention in order to reduce the need for accident management.

Our goal is to help you become a better diver and buddy.

Be Ready for Your Journey

All our specialty courses are based on our signature training method — the SSI Diver Diamond. To become a comfortable and confident diver, it takes four ingredients:

Proper Knowledge

As in all SSI training programs, knowledge is power and replaces fears and fantasies with correct information. In this program, you will acquire the specific knowledge related to the Diver Stress & Rescue Specialty.

Proper Skills

Repetition is the mother of all skills. Under the guidance of your SSI Dive Professional, you will learn the specific skills and techniques needed to recognize stress and stay in control of the situation.

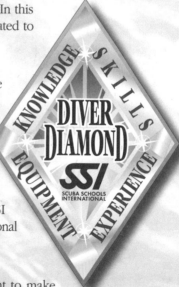

Proper Equipment

The safest way to dive is in your own personally fitted Total Diving System. For this and all SSI Continuing Education courses, you may need additional equipment to perform a rescue.

Proper Experience

Gaining the knowledge, skills and equipment to make advanced dives is only one part of the journey. Going diving is the only way you can gain the actual experience needed to become a comfortable and confident diver.

How Far Do You Want to Go?

If you believe the journey is just as important as the destination, then SSI's Continuing Education is for you. Taking specialties is a great way to hone your skills and learn some new ones. Continuing Education is exciting and limitless. It is your chance to begin exploring beyond the surface. Choose your personal combination of training and diving experience to reach your diving goals today!

SSI's Continuing Education courses are all menu-based home study programs. These specialty courses are designed so that you can learn at your own pace when it's convenient for you. Menu-based means you can take courses in a combined manner or one at a time based on your personal interest. Simply choose from specialties like, Photography, Enriched Air Nitrox, Wreck, Navigation, Night & Limited Visibility and you're on your way.

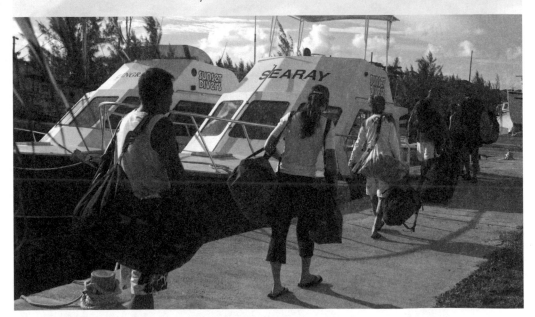

Getting involved is easy! If you're not sure which specialties you want to try, sign up for the Advanced Adventurer program. You will be able to take 5 dives and try 5 different specialties. Upon completion you will be recognized with an Advanced Adventurer card. These dives also count towards your rating if you choose to continue your training in one of the specialty areas covered.

For detailed information regarding SSI Specialty programs ask your SSI Dive Center or visit www.diveSSI.com

Intro

5 OR MORE LOGGED DIVES

LEVEL OF EXPERIENCE: 1

Complete the SSI Open Water Diver course & get this card!

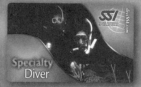

12 OR MORE LOGGED DIVES

LEVEL OF EXPERIENCE: 2

Complete Level 2 dives & 2 Specialty Courses.

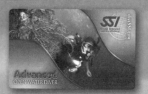

24 OR MORE LOGGED DIVES

LEVEL OF EXPERIENCE: 3

Complete Level 3 dives & 4 Specialty Courses.

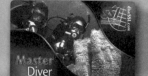

50 OR MORE LOGGED DIVES

LEVEL OF EXPERIENCE: 4

Complete Level 4 dives, 4 Specialty Courses & the Diver Stress & Rescue Course.

AVAILABLE SPECIALTIES — *Take one or take them all!*

- ◇ Adaptive Scuba Diving
- ◇ Boat Diving
- ◇ Computer Diving
- ◇ Deep Diving
- ◇ Digital Underwater Photography
- ◇ Diver Stress & Rescue
- ◇ Dry Suit Diving
- ◇ Emergency Training
  - – First Aid & CPR
  - – Emergency Oxygen
  - – AED
  - – Bloodborne Pathogens
- ◇ Enriched Air Nitrox
- ◇ Equipment Techniques

- ◇ Navigation
- ◇ Night and Limited Visibility Diving
- ◇ Perfect Buoyancy
- ◇ Science of Diving
- ◇ Search & Recovery
- ◇ Technical Extended Range
  - – Advanced Nitrox
  - – Technical Foundations
  - – Decompression Procedures
  - – Advanced Decompression
  - – Normoxic Trimix
- ◇ Waves, Tides & Currents
- ◇ Wreck Diving

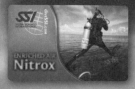

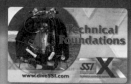

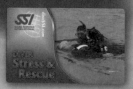

You can become a Dive Leader once you have completed Level 4! Ask your SSI Dive Center for complete details.

Instructor Levels
Quality Divers Start with Qualified Instructors

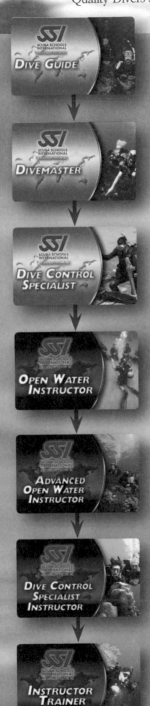

Other Instructor Programs
◆ Specialty Instructor
◆ Diver Stress & Rescue Instructor
◆ Enriched Air Nitrox Instructor
◆ Scuba Rangers Instructor
◆ Technical Extended Range
  – Advanced Nitrox Instructor
  – Technical Foundations Instructor
  – Decompression Procedures Instructor
  – Advanced Decompression Procedures Instructor
  – Normoxic Trimix Instructor
  – TechXR Instructor Trainer

REWARDS FOR EXPERIENCE
No Training Required!

Taking a specific number of specialties and continuing your pursuit of dives allows you to earn higher rating levels. SSI Ratings are the only ratings in the industry that combine training and experience requirements, proving that SSI Ratings are truly earned.

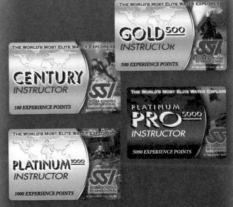

Reward yourself as you reach new milestones in your diving adventures!

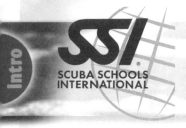

About SSI

Scuba Schools International grew out of the passion of a few avid divers who were intent on making it possible for anyone to learn to scuba dive.

SSI provides education materials, dive training and scuba certification for divers, dive instructors, dive centers and dive resorts around the world. Since 1970, SSI has expanded to 27 International Offices, doing business in 110 countries with training materials in 25 languages representing over 2,400 dive centers and resorts. SSI Certification Cards are welcomed all over the planet, wherever you choose to dive.

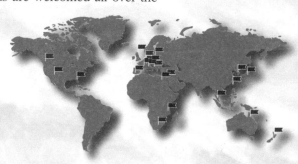

Scuba Schools International is clearly a name you can trust in the diving community and we attribute that success to uncompromising standards and a focus on quality not quantity.

Involvement

As well as being an industry leader, SSI is also a founding member of the industry's standards body in the USA and abroad – in the USA, it's the RSTC (Recreational Scuba Training Council) and in Europe, it's the WRSTC and the EU (European Standards – EN 14153-1-3 for divers and 144413-1-2 for scuba instructors).

Reward Yourself. You Deserve it.

Becoming certified in Diver Stress & Rescue is an achievement. Be sure to reward yourself for reaching this major milestone with an SSI Diver Stress & Rescue Diving certification card. This is an opportunity to commemorate your hard-earned accomplishment.

Where to Go From Here.

We are certain that your journey through Diver Stress & Rescue will be everything you imagined and more. Don't forget you can always combine other specialties to increase your diving knowledge — the possibilities are limitless. Now, let's go have some fun!

Intro

Introduction to Diver Stress & Rescue

Scuba diving is an exciting, challenging and rewarding experience. This activity continues to grow year after year as more and more people are enticed into the underwater world. Young people as well as older men and women are now enjoying an activity that was once dominated by young, strong men. People from all aspects of life are finding scuba diving to be a social activity, and one which offers some of the most spectacular scenery they have ever witnessed.

As the diversity among divers grows, those divers still need to make a personal commitment to the sport, for their benefit and their buddy's. The basics of being a relaxed and competent diver are the proper use of equipment, comfortable performance of basic skills, and experience. In addition, divers can learn about taking precautions against dive-related anxieties, helping their buddies, and preparing for the accidents that can occur.

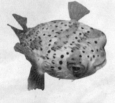

Diver stress is the unwelcome result of a lack of experience or the failure to take necessary precautions. Stress and the resulting feeling of panic are largely responsible for the drop-out rate in scuba, as well as many diving accidents. Case studies show that these accidents are related to cardiovascular disease, lack of training for the dives being conducted, inexperience, exhaustion, panic and rapid ascents. The result of serious accidents is usually air embolism, decompression sickness, and drowning.

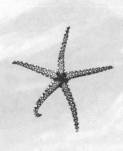

Ironically, these problems are in most cases preventable, with the exception of cardiovascular disease, just by identifying stress and its cause. Recognition of stress and then dealing with it, as covered in the first three chapters, will help you and your buddy avoid the need to be rescued or becoming the victim of a diving accident.

Intro

Rescue skills are, of course, very important and must be learned, as well as how to manage an accident situation. These are covered in Chapters 4 through 6 of this text. Even if you know how to keep yourself out of emergency situations, it is possible you will be at the scene of one someday. Knowing what to do may help save another diver's life.

In the SSI *Diver Stress & Rescue* course, you will first analyze what causes stress, and then what causes diver stress in particular. We will then discuss how a normal dive turns into a rescue situation and, more important, how to help prevent that from happening in the first place.

Knowing first aid and CPR are vital to managing a diving accident effectively, and are also valuable in everyday life. Your local SSI Dive Center may offer First Aid and CPR courses or know where you can receive equivalent training. In order to receive your SSI *Diver Stress & Rescue* certification card, you must be current in CPR and first aid.

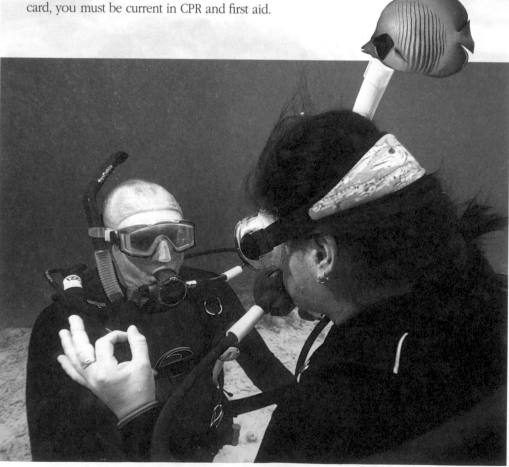

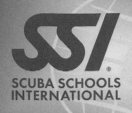

PART 1
Stress

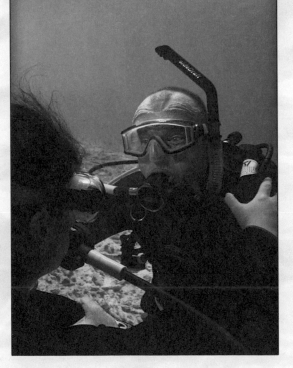

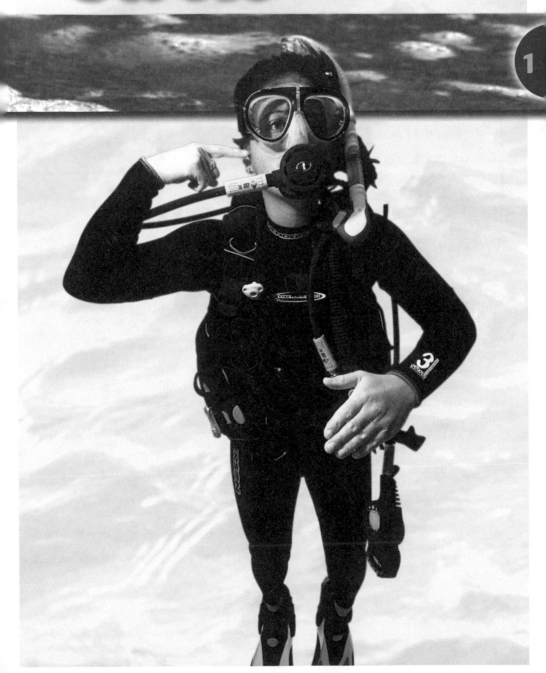

Stress

For most of us, stress has become part of our daily lives. Since stress has come to be associated with hypertension and other medical problems, researchers are continuously inventing ways for us to deal with it, and we are responding to these recommendations with better dietary and exercise habits in our daily routines.

Section 1 Objectives
After completing this section you will be able to:

♦ List the three factors of STRESS that determine whether it is positive or negative,

♦ State the fight-or-flight syndrome,

♦ Understand the vulnerability of stress,

♦ Describe the psycho-respiratory cycle.

What is Stress?

Stress has been described as the result of pressures or demands which outweigh a person's ability or capacity to respond to them. Stress can be detected at any point as it develops — by you or by another who is close by — and the earlier it is detected, the easier it is to respond to.

Stress Can Be Good?

Some stress can actually be quite useful. It can be a simple warning sign which will alert you to do something about a particular demand. A consistent but low level of stress is healthy because it keeps us alert and warns us of danger. There is also truth to the claim that certain people "work better under pressure."

Everyone has a different tolerance for stress, so it can, therefore, be either positive or negative. According to Georgia Witkin-Lanoil, whether stress is positive or negative is determined by three factors[1]:

1. **Your sense of choice:** A chosen demand is a stimulation. The stimulation is sought for the sake of thrill or adventure. Or, in the case of someone taking on a productive challenge, it facilitates the feeling of

[1]Georgia Witkin-Lanoil, *The Male Stress Syndrome* (New Yourk: New Market, 1986), p. 25

working better under pressure. Demands that are not chosen create undesired pressure and negative stress.

2. **Your degree of control:** As your real or perceived control over a situation diminishes, your real or perceived stress increases.

> Stress multiplies if a demand overpowers your ability to maintain control over the situation.

3. **Your ability to anticipate the consequences:** Adaptation and adjustment are most difficult when demands and outcomes are not predictable. The unexpected and unknown create negative stress.

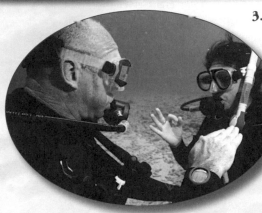

One buddy can usually stay in control during a stress situation.

It is easy to imagine the inherent positive stress of diving (relying on mental acuity and equipment for safety) turning into negative stress. The underwater environment can be full of surprises and can present situations that you must be ready for, such as the loss of your mask or a leg cramp. If you are unable to anticipate such situations, your sense of control will be threatened.

Though it is impossible to be "ready" for a surprise, the trick is to consciously recognize a new demand and to respond to it calmly and logically. Learning to detect and control stress will come with experience, and with the consistent awareness that demands may arise — this awareness fitting into the category of positive stress.

The Buddy System

One of the best arguments in favor of always using the buddy system is the improbability of both divers becoming stressed to the point of losing control at the same time. In a stress situation there will almost always be at least one diver who maintains control and is able to lend aid.

KNOWLEDGE • SKILLS • EQUIPMENT • EXPERIENCE
DIVER DIAMOND
SSI
SCUBA SCHOOLS INTERNATIONAL

The Stress Response

Stress is human

Stress is a very human response to the kind of arousal and excitement which starts the flow of adrenaline. The sudden stimulus we feel when frightened, startled, or threatened is called the fight-or-flight syndrome. The flight-or-fight response developed in early humans as a means of survival. It gave them the sense to run from danger or to fight if trapped.

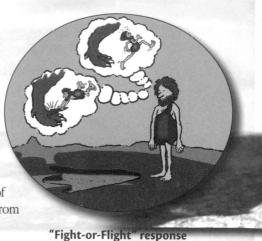

"Fight-or-Flight" response in early humans.

Modern humans have a keenly developed fight-or-flight response. Some of us may have experienced a rush of adrenaline before doing something as non-life-threatening as asking for a raise. Whether you are a nervous personality who is overly sensitive to stress or a more relaxed type who seems to stay calm under adverse circumstances, recognizing the signs of stress is the first step in learning to control it and respond to it logically. Early warning signs include:

- Warm, or flushed complexion
- Perspiration
- Stomach "butterflies" or nausea
- Rapid heartbeat
- Shortness of breath
- Muscle tension

These signs occur by instinct. When the signs occur, stop and think. Identify the source. While diving it may be the simple matter of a difficulty with maintaining neutral buoyancy, which would be easy to identify and resolve. Unless it is handled at this point, however, your stress level may increase due to the introduction of a new stressor — your lack of buoyancy control may separate you from your buddy, for instance. Or, if you are preoccupied by a pinch in your wet suit, you may not be prepared when you catch your cylinder valve in fishing line. It is the combinations of stressors that can threaten your control.

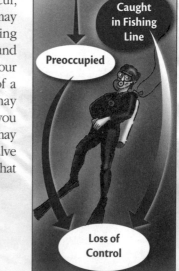

Wet Suit Squeeze

Caught in Fishing Line

Preoccupied

Loss of Control

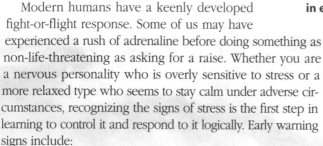

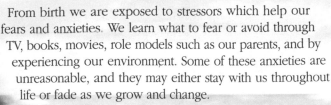

Stress is Learned

From birth we are exposed to stressors which help our fears and anxieties. We learn what to fear or avoid through TV, books, movies, role models such as our parents, and by experiencing our environment. Some of these anxieties are unreasonable, and they may either stay with us throughout life or fade as we grow and change.

Bad experiences such as falling from a tree, burning a hand on a stove, or being injured in an auto accident might teach us to avoid situations known to cause pain or threaten our survival.

Children may fail to learn how to make important decisions for themselves when they are forced to lead a sheltered life, and others consistently make those decisions for them. Naturally, some of these children grow up to be irresponsible adults. If a diver with this behavior pattern were to become separated from his or her buddy, a sudden sense of aloneness might trigger negative stress.

Stress is Social

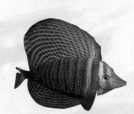

Anxieties which cause stress come not only from childhood experiences, but also from social behaviors. We learn what is socially permissible, and through this we gain a sense of ourselves and how to interact with others. Fear is a powerful emotion which can be disguised in many forms, including social forms such as embarrassment or reluctance.

Realizing that no one is immune to fear is a step toward being better able to manage stress in a social situation.

Fear of failure is a strong stressor. Some learn to accept failure as a part of learning, but others may develop performance anxiety or the inability to perform when the act may be socially scrutinized. Divers sometimes feel they should be able to dive in any situation, even though their experience level doesn't allow it. Just being certified doesn't mean you are qualified for any diving situation you will encounter.

1

Another social fear is looking bad in front of others. We all try to avoid embarrassment, but this can be dangerous if, for example, we are too embarrassed to admit we've forgotten how to perform a certain skill. We must learn how to admit a lack of knowledge, or admit when we are in need of assistance, for everyone is in need of assistance at some time.

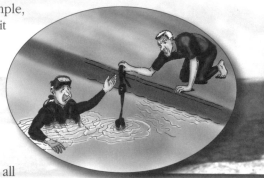

Stress is Personal

Although there may be stressors we all share in common, many vary by individual. Good buddy communication and attention to your dive objectives in the pre-dive phase will help prevent initial anxieties, and prevent the stress of going ahead with someone else's plans even though you are uncomfortable with them.

An embarrassing situation can create stress

A critical skill in diving is learning how to dive within your limits, and to "know when to say when."

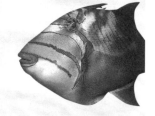

Willingness to take risks varies from individual to individual, too. Most people enjoy a certain level of risk. It can be fun. But others are at opposite extremes: some avoid risk at all costs, and others seek it earnestly. It is important to realize where you fit in, because if you engage in risk beyond your capacity to remain in control, great stress can result. If you are the non-risk taker, it is quite possible to enjoy diving at a safe, comfortable pace and avoid stress. If you are the thrill seeker, it is necessary for you to realize that taking extreme risks while diving can lead to danger.

Who is Vulnerable to Stress

There seem to be certain types of people who are more prone to stress based on their coping style. For the purpose of this text, we have divided these people into two categories: anxious-dependent and competitive-perfectionist. Although these two personalities may seem opposite by nature, they are each uniquely susceptible to stress.

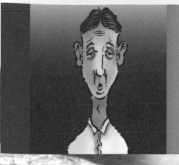

Anxious-dependents

Anxious-dependents are susceptible to stress because they often lack control over themselves, are often nervous, and depend a great deal on others for help and guidance. They lack self-confidence, fear stimulus, often feel helpless, and often are poor in health and lack physical conditioning.

Anxious-dependents should learn to dive with more than one buddy because this helps them to learn while preventing the "easy out" of depending on one person entirely. Through confidence building, proper training, and practice these people can become proficient divers, but must first recognize and face their own susceptibility to stress.

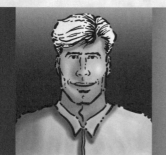

Competitive-perfectionist

The *competitive-perfectionist*, on the other hand, is aggressive and appears to be in control at all times. Persons displaying this personality type may actually be "born to greatness," or may instead be covering up inner anxieties. Competitive-perfectionists desire risk and challenge, have difficulty in asking for or accepting assistance, and are very concerned with public approval.

These behaviors can spell trouble in situations which pose possible hazards. Competitive-perfectionists are likely to hide their need for help. In diving this not only endangers themselves, but also their buddies. For perfectionists there is only success or failure, and "failure" is the result of a task not performed to their own strict standards. What such people must realize is that perfection is relative, and is also unobtainable. The price of the stress created in trying to obtain it is not worth the imagined prize.

Scuba diving is not a challenge to be won or lost, it is an activity that provides pleasure and enjoyment to the participant.

The Psycho-Respiratory Cycle

Whereas stress is the result of a lack of experience, panic is an overpowering fear caused by a real or imagined loss of control over a situation. After initial stress occurs, there is normally a common sequence of events that occurs prior to the onset of panic. By being aware of these events, you can begin to understand how stress can multiply into panic and how to stop it.

It begins with any of a number of stressors which create an increased energy demand on the diver. The increased energy demand leads to an increase in respiratory and heart rates. This energy/respiration/heart rate demand causes anxiety when combined with the original stressor. This is known as the *psycho-respiratory cycle*.

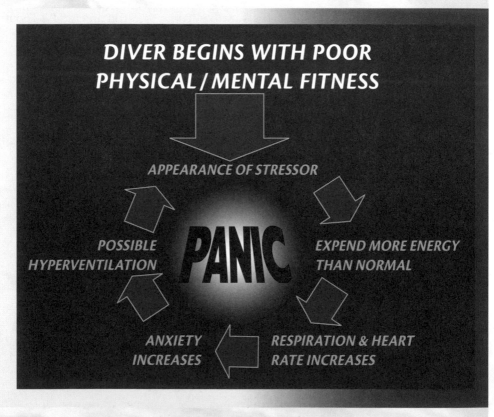

DIVER BEGINS WITH POOR PHYSICAL / MENTAL FITNESS

APPEARANCE OF STRESSOR

EXPEND MORE ENERGY THAN NORMAL

RESPIRATION & HEART RATE INCREASES

ANXIETY INCREASES

POSSIBLE HYPERVENTILATION

PANIC

The Psycho-Respiratory Cycle.

If a stressor such as a strong current is present, the unexpected occurrence of an additional stressor, such as the appearance of a dangerous animal, may further accelerate the respiration rate until the diver experiences a carbon dioxide buildup. If the cycle goes too far, hyperventilation can result, causing the diver to feel as if he or she is suffocating, which under water would nearly always result in panic or at least a dangerous rush to the surface.

By being aware of the cycle, you can beat it at any time. Simply stop, rest, assess the causes, and take actions to alleviate them. If it is something you cannot control, abort the dive. By breathing deeply and relaxing, you can get your breathing under control and stop the psycho-respiratory cycle.

Now that we've discussed stress and who may or may not be susceptible to it, you should understand the importance of recognizing stress in yourself. If you are truthful about your present ability to manage stress, you can begin to learn how to become less effected by it, which in the long run will increase your diving comfort.

Let's go on in Section 2 to look more specifically at the causes of stress in diving and how to prevent it from occurring.

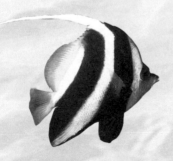

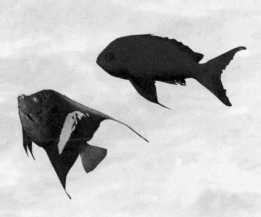

Section 1 Review Questions

1. Stress has been described as the result of pressures or demands which outweigh a person's _____ or _____ to respond to them.

2. A consistent but low level of stress is _____ because it keeps us _____ and _____ us of danger.

3. Everyone has a different tolerance for stress, so it can, therefore, be either _____ or _____ .

4. Demands that are not chosen create undesired _____ and _____ stress.

5. Stress multiplies if a _____ overpowers your ability to maintain _____ over the situation.

6. The unexpected and unknown create _____ _____ .

7. Learning to _____ and _____ stress will come with _____ , and with the consistent awareness that demands may arise — this awareness fitting into the category of positive stress.

8. The sudden stimulus we feel when frightened, startled, or threatened is called the _____ or _____ _____ .

9. Early warning signs of stress include: (List two)

_____

_____

10. It is the _____ of stressors that can threaten your control.

11. We all try to avoid _____ , but this can be dangerous if, for example, we are too _____ to admit we've forgotten how to perform a certain skill.

12. A critical skill in diving is learning how to dive within your limits, and to " _____ _____ _____

_____ _____ ."

13. _____ – _____ are susceptible to stress because they often lack control over themselves, are often nervous, and depend a great deal on others for help and guidance.

14. The _____ – _____ , on the other hand, is aggressive and appears to be in control at all times.

15. Whereas stress is the result of a lack of _____ , _____ is an overpowering fear caused by a real or imagined loss of control over a situation.

Stress in Diving — Causes & Prevention

2

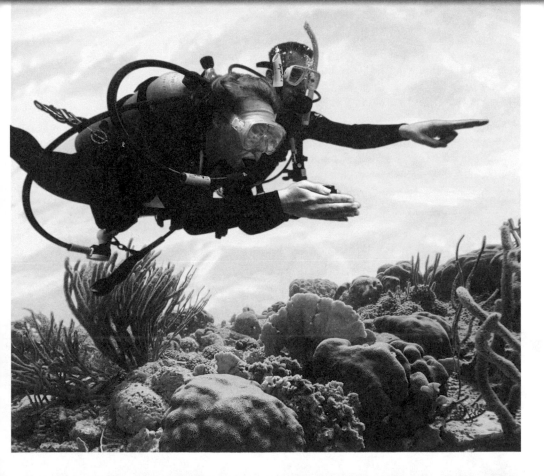

In order to relieve or prevent stress you must first be able to identify its source. If you understand the various causes of stress in diving, you'll be able to avoid these situations or know how to deal with them should they arise.

Section 2 Objectives
After completing this section you will be able to:

◆ State the physical and psychological causes of stress as they relate to diving,

◆ Describe the environment- and equipment-related causes of stress,

◆ Understand how proper training and skills can help in avoiding excess stress.

Stress usually originates in divers because of five reasons: Physical causes, Psychological causes, Equipment problems, Environmental conditions, or Lack of skill.

Some stress-producing situations are unpredictable, but others are functions of our own personal preparedness. Being healthy, having the proper skills, and using good quality and well-maintained equipment will help you stay a step ahead of stress.

Physical Causes

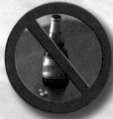

A healthy body functions better under water and allows you to dive for longer periods of time more comfortably. In addition, a healthy body usually harbors a sharper mind, a mind that can foresee problems or respond to them quickly if they do occur. If, for example, we are out of shape or drink too much, chances are that in the water we will experience fatigue more readily than someone who is physically prepared for the demanding activity that diving can be. Poor health and bad dive decisions that affect the body can inevitably lead to discomfort and therefore to stress.

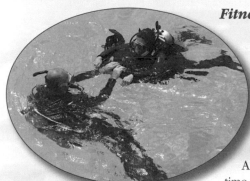

Fitness

Poor physical fitness will make you more susceptible to fatigue and various mental stressors. Divers who are not physically fit may have a difficult time with the physical activity of putting on and taking off equipment, and with the physical exertion required in diving. An unfit person may also have a hard time assisting or rescuing a buddy in need.

This is why exercise and a good diet should be part of a diver's ongoing fitness plan. A well-balanced diet consisting of complex carbohydrates such as whole grains, rice, fruit, and vegetables will help your body function better under water. As a rule of thumb, if you are sick, don't dive. Before diving, if you require medication, get the approval of a medical physician versed in diving. Also, never second guess, even if you feel you are in excellent health.

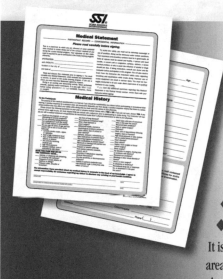

Get a medical checkup each diving season, and be especially conscientious if you are over 45 and have one or more of the following conditions:

◆ Currently smoke a pipe, cigars or cigarettes

◆ Are overweight and/or out of shape

◆ Are taking regular medication

◆ Have high cholesterol and/or a family history of heart attack and strokes

◆ Have had recent surgery or illness

◆ Have asthma, epilepsy, or other respiratory problems

It is strongly recommended that you find a physician in your area who dives. A diving physician will naturally know more about the aspects of diving which can affect your health.

Lastly, medical experts agree that women who are pregnant, or who suspect they are pregnant, should not dive. For other medical concerns, call the Divers Alert Network in the U.S., or the Divers Emergency Service in the Pacific for more details.

Fatigue

Driving several hours to a dive site, staying up too late, feeling ill, and a variety of other circumstances, alone or combined, can create fatigue. Diving requires a clear mind and a fresh body. Do not dive when overly fatigued, especially if other factors are present which could contribute to fatigue — such as diving in cold water.

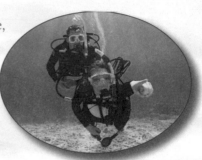

Fatigue is most likely to occur at the end of a dive, especially if you have to deal with currents on your way back to an exit point, or if you have been called upon to perform too many mental tasks during your dive or dive day. Monitor yourself and buddy for fatigue throughout the day, being ready to abort before exhaustion strikes.

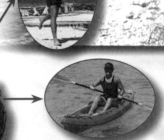

Open water diving does not require superior athletic prowess, but it does require cardiovascular efficiency. Cardiovascular fitness can usually be maintained through a minimum three to four thirty-minute aerobic workouts per week. If you have not been exercising on a regular basis, it is advisable that you get a checkup before starting your fitness plan.

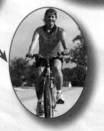

In addition to aerobic exercise such as jogging, swimming, and cycling, strength conditioning will give you more stamina for long swims against currents, for hauling heavy dive equipment, and will prepare you for an emergency such as a buddy rescue.

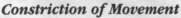

As a general rule, a diver should be fit enough to respond to an emergency without becoming exhausted or risking heart failure. This indicates a level of fitness beyond fundamental sufficiency for scuba diving.

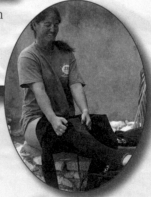

Constriction of Movement

Wearing equipment that is too small will constrict your ability to move freely, making you feel awkward and exert excess energy. It can also restrict

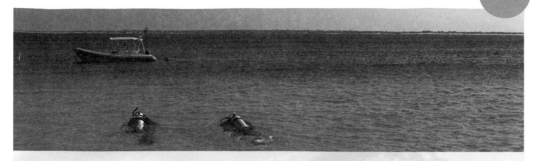

your breathing and circulation, causing you to become cold faster and to use up energy sooner.

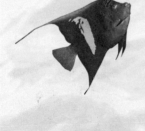

Buddies

Having a buddy and being a buddy are closely related to another major objective of any dive; being prepared and, consequently, avoiding stress.

Movement can also be constricted by entanglement, or entrapment in confined areas. Entanglement in kelp or fishing line is not serious and can be managed with a diver's tool and the assistance of a buddy. Entrapment in caves, wrecks, or under ice is very serious and can lead to panic. Your buddy is there to help you out of potential danger, but only if you remain under control. Always dive with a buddy, wear complete, proper-fitting, and high quality equipment, and be aware of hazards when diving in wrecks, caves and ice. Avoid these situations altogether unless you have the proper equipment and extensive specialty training.

Cold Water and Hypothermia

Cold water can affect both your mental and bodily functions, possibly preventing clear thinking and restricting normal physical activity. It is uncomfortable and can be painful, and puts a strain on your body as you try to warm-up. Severely cold water can also cause equipment malfunction. By definition, water below 70°F/21°C is considered cold, due to the fact that body heat is absorbed twenty-five times faster in water than air.

Hypothermia occurs when the body's core temperature drops below its normal 98.6°F/37°C. The lower the body temperature drops, the more danger the diver is in. Symptoms of hypothermia include confusion, bluing of the skin, rigidity, uncontrollable shivering, and loss of coordination. All hypothermia victims should be warmed, and severe hypothermics should be warmed by qualified medical personnel only. Improper warming can cause complications.

To avoid the effects of cold water and hypothermia, wear the proper exposure suit for the water temperature at the depth you will be diving, not just the surface temperature. Add a hood and gloves to prevent heat loss through the head, and stop your dive if you begin to get uncomfortably cold. SSI recommends using a dry suit in water colder than 65°F/18°C.

It is recommended that if you dive in a dry suit, you participate in an SSI Dry Suit specialty course. Check with your SSI Dive Center on the availability of a Dry Suit specialty course.

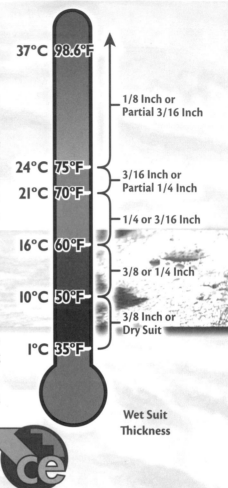

37°C 98.6°F

1/8 Inch or Partial 3/16 Inch

24°C 75°F
21°C 70°F

3/16 Inch or Partial 1/4 Inch

1/4 or 3/16 Inch

16°C 60°F

3/8 or 1/4 Inch

10°C 50°F

3/8 Inch or Dry Suit

1°C 35°F

Wet Suit Thickness

Psychological Causes

Some stressors are attributed to a lack of mental preparedness, mental control, and mental coping. When a buddy show signs of mental unpreparedness or vulnerability, he or she will probably not be aware of it, while you will be. If you yourself are susceptible to such stressors, learn to avoid them through better preparation and control. Experience is probably the best prescription for most psychological anxieties related to diving.

Anyone can experience stress, and most healthy individuals are capable of panicking under extreme duress; but regardless of these ever-present possibilities, divers should be comfortable in the water. Persons prone to panic behavior should not dive. Psychological contraindications to diving include active psychosis, depression, claustrophobia, drug

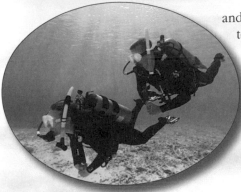

Buddies add pleasure as well as safety to the diving experience.

and/or alcohol abuse, proneness to panic attack, and the use of psychotropic medication.

Poor Judgment

Poor judgment plays a part in any diving accident, whether because of ignorance or inexperience. Diving beyond your limits, diving without proper equipment, diving in poor weather conditions, and diving while ill or fatigued can all contribute to stress. Starting a dive with a partial cylinder of air, diving in high surface waves, and failing to take an extra light on a night dive all can lead to problems.

If you use good judgment, dive within your limits, and are prepared with the proper equipment, you should be able to avoid stress and have a gratifying experience.

Nervousness

A diver may be nervous for a variety of reasons (new equipment, unfamiliar conditions/location), but the reassurance of a caring buddy can make for a safe and enjoyable dive for both parties.

Buddy System Failure

Both diving without a buddy and failing to communicate with your buddy can be stressful. Imagine finding yourself in need of help and it is not available. If your buddy seems nervous or anxious, constant communication through hand signals, physical contact, and eye contact will provide encouragement.

The buddy system has become a worldwide standard among the diving community. Buddies add pleasure as well as safety to the diving experience. They also lend a hand in making small gear adjustments, providing emergency assistance, and getting emergency help if necessary. More importantly they provide psychological reassurance through communication, and just by being present. Many times in a stressful situation all that is needed is a reassuring pat on the back.

A good buddy team depends on proper matching. Buddies with like interests, abilities, and objectives should be paired together. One exception to this is the need to pair a diver lacking confidence with one who is experienced and can assist and emotionally support the novice. Also, friends and spouses who are incompatible as divers may be better off diving with other partners.

There are a few basic things buddies can do while diving to assure confidence. Work as a team — constantly communicating, monitoring each other's actions, and providing support when needed. Always stay within sight of each other, and if visibility is low, establish physical contact such as holding hands. In order to facilitate visual contact and communication, swim side-by-side, not one behind the other.

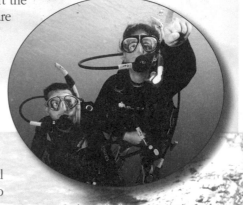

Swim side-by-side to facilitate communication.

Drugs and Alcohol

It is recommended that you get a medical opinion from a diving physician before using any drugs, prescription or otherwise. The use of controlled substances is discouraged because of their ability to impair judgment and affect alertness and other mental faculties. In addition, the side effects of drugs combined with pressure are not known, so even commonly used drugs may affect people adversely.

Alcohol should not be abused the night before a dive, should not be used during a dive, and should be used in moderation at all other times.

Alcohol can reduce your tolerance for high pressure nitrogen, which can make you more susceptible to nitrogen narcosis. Drinking alcohol before and between dives can also prevent nitrogen from quickly entering and exiting blood because of reduced circulation, making divers more at risk for decompression sickness. If you should decide to indulge in alcohol the night before, avoid diving the following day.

Equipment-Related Causes

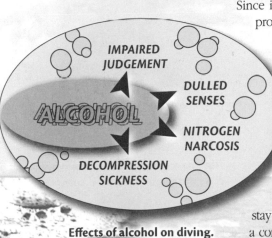

Effects of alcohol on diving.

Since it is a much more common problem than running out of air, equipment misuse may be the single largest contributor to stress. Too much weight, a wet suit that fits improperly, a BC that is too large or small, fins that are too loose, or a leaky mask can lead to increases in stress.

For example, if you are negatively buoyant and must fight to stay off the bottom, plus your mask has a continuous leak, you may be "on edge" and distracted. You may begin to breathe a little faster, then your heart rate accelerates, and you find yourself experiencing stress. Simply making sure your equipment fits well, is correctly adjusted, and you know how to use it properly will virtually eliminate equipment-related stress.

The importance of a high quality Total Diving System which works and fits properly cannot be overemphasized. Since scuba diving depends on equipment, you can guess that many of the anxieties divers experience originate with poorly maintained or misused equipment. Your Total Diving System is your lifeline to the deep. Take care of it and it will take care of you.

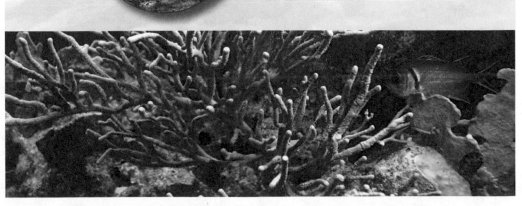

Equipment Loss

The unexpected loss of equipment during a dive can contribute to a loss of control, especially when other stressors such as fatigue are already present. We can function temporarily without equipment, such as a fin, mask, or light, but only if we remain in control and act quickly and calmly to replace it. If it is lost and cannot be retrieved, abort the dive; it is unsafe to dive without all necessary equipment — even if it is possible. Your buddy can help you retrieve and replace lost equipment or surface without it. Most importantly, never begin a dive without a complete set of equipment including: Mask, Fins, Snorkel, Exposure Suit, Cylinder, BC, Power Inflator, Regulator, Alternate Air Source, Depth Gauge, Pressure Gauge, Timing Device, Compass and Knife. Also, add any special equipment required for the particular type of diving you are engaging in, such as plenty of lights for night diving.

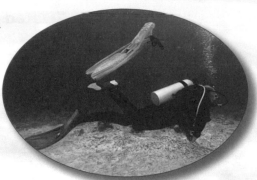

The unexpected loss of equipment can contribute to a loss of control.

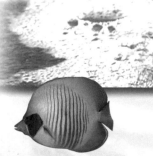

Equipment Maintenance

The use of a properly maintained Total Diving System enhances the enjoyment and overall safety of the sport. Nearly all equipment-related stress involves not having the right equipment, poorly maintained equipment, or ill-fitting equipment; there is little risk of accident when using new or well-maintained equipment. It is important to check your equipment before leaving for your dive destination, and it is recommended that cylinders and first- and second-stage regulators be inspected and serviced at least annually.

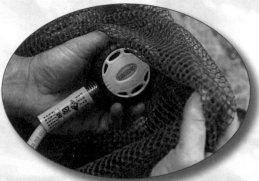

There is little risk of accident when using new or well-maintained equipment.

To check your equipment, assemble the scuba unit where you have access to a tank of water — a bathtub is adequate. Before turning on your air, check the second-stage regulator by exhaling through it; if you cannot exhale, the exhaust valve

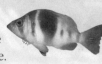

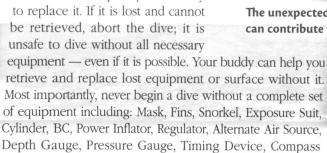

may be stuck shut and will need repair. Then, dry-breathe from the mouthpiece; you should not be able to inhale. If you can, there is something faulty in the system that will need correction. Next, turn the air on and check your hoses for cracks and leaks; inflate and deflate the BC in water to check it for leaks.

Many manufacturers require annual maintenance to keep warranties in effect. Be sure you know what manufacturers' requirements are, and make certain your equipment — especially life support equipment — is serviced by a qualified technician. Manufacturers are continually upgrading equipment to make it safer, more comfortable, and easier to use. It is not only a good idea, but it is also safer to follow these developments and replace your old equipment.

The SSI Equipment Service Program

The Equipment Service Program, which is available through your SSI Dive Center, is a complete maintenance program designed to keep the components of your Total Diving System performing to the best of their potential. Below is an explanation of each of the services that make up the SSI Equipment Service Program.

Air Delivery System Protection

Regulators are totally disassembled and cleaned in a special cleaning solution. High-pressure and low-pressure seats are replaced along with all dynamic o-rings, exhaust valves, and high-pressure filters. Performance tests are conducted to manufacturer warranty specifications.

Nitrox Air Delivery System Protection

This is the same as Air Delivery System Protection, but is performed on Nitrox equipment. A green Nitrox hose sleeve is used to mark your Nitrox Air Delivery System rather than a yellow hose sleeve.

Information System Protection

Submersible pressure gauges, depth gauges, pressure activated dive timers, and dive computers are checked for accuracy in a pressure vessel, and the indicated readings versus true readings are noted.

Buoyancy Control System Protection

Buoyancy compensators are inspected for leaks, buckle strap tension and bladder seam integrity. Inflator mechanisms are disassembled, cleaned and rebuilt, the inner bladder rinsed with B.C. conditioner and over-pressure release valves are cleaned and tested for proper operation, all to manufacturer warranty specifications.

Visual Inspection Protection (and Visual Plus®)

Annually, cylinders are inspected internally and externally for rust, corrosion and cracks to the standards of DOT and CGA. It is suggested that aluminium cylinders be tested with Visual Plus to ensure the integrity and strength of the neck and threads.

Exposure System Protection

Services are available for exposure suits (wet and dry). Minor repairs are done in-house and alterations are done with the original manufacturer.

Keep track of all your repairs and servicing in an equipment maintenance schedule such as the one provided in the back of your SSI Log Book. When you have your equipment serviced or repaired, take along your SSI Total DiveLog so the technician can record the service. This will be valuable should you decide to upgrade your equipment someday.

Failure to Monitor the Information System

Running low on air or out of air under water is one of the most stressful situations a diver can experience. When air is suddenly lost, the natural instinct is to rush to the surface — a very dangerous thing to do. Failure to monitor the pressure gauge is the main reason people run out of air, whether it's failing to confirm your cylinder is full before entering the water, or failing to check the gauge periodically throughout the dive.

When diving in either extremely clear or murky water it is hard to estimate depth visually. So it's important to monitor your computer or depth gauge regularly, and

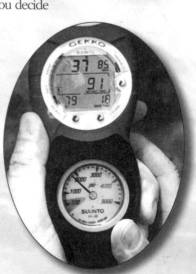

Failure to monitor the pressure gauge is the main reason people run out of air.

as an extra safety precaution make a safety stop at 15 feet/5 metres for three to five minutes on every dive.

Failure to monitor your direction or time can also lead to stress. By not monitoring where you are going or how long you have been down, you may end up a long way from your ascent point without enough air for the return trip. Not using a compass will result in constantly having to surface for orientation, or in a long, exhausting surface swim to your exit point.

Monitoring your Information System does not need to be an all-consuming effort; an occasional glance to find out the status on your depth, pressure, time, and direction is all that is needed. If you have a computer, you will also want to monitor it for your no-decompression safety margins. By sticking to your planned depth and time you should be able to avoid decompression sickness, by monitoring your direction you should be able to easily find your exit point, and by monitoring your pressure gauge you should never run low on air. Your Information System is designed for your safety, but only when it is monitored.

Environmental Causes

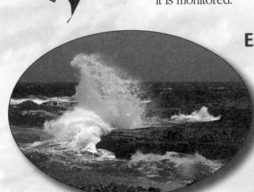

Being well-trained, well-equipped, and even highly experienced does not necessarily qualify a diver as "safe." No matter how educated the diver is, if a bad decision about where, when, or under what conditions the dive is made, even an experienced diver can get into trouble. Overconfidence does not qualify you to dive in unfamiliar conditions, and continued experience does not necessarily mean you should take greater and greater risks as a diver. Always dive when weather and conditions permit, and dive in specialty situations only if you are qualified in that particular specialty.

Cancel, postpone, or abort dives involving potentially hazardous conditions.

Poor Environmental Conditions

Poor environmental conditions, especially when combined with another cause of stress such as fatigue, can spell danger. Low visibility, currents, surface chop, storms, and excessively cold water are but a few of the environmental conditions that can cause stress when diving. The underwater world, whether an inland lake or an ocean, can be powerful and intimidating. A day that begins with good conditions can turn bad during your dive, so you must be prepared to adapt to whatever arises.

Whenever necessary, cancel, postpone, or abort a dive that involves potentially hazardous environmental conditions.

There will always be another diving day or another diving vacation, do not take an unnecessary risk when there are plenty of good diving days left in your future.

Unfamiliar Diving

Unfamiliar diving conditions are those in which you have no experience or training. It goes without saying that you should not dive unless properly trained, but diving situations vary and are not always ones for which specialty training is required. For instance, if you are used to boat diving and you're about to do a shore dive for the first time, you will not be familiar with the entry and exit required in these conditions, nor will you be prepared for the actions of localized currents, such as a rip current.

As discussed earlier, an inability to predict consequences and a loss of control can cause stress, which can lead to panic. Diving locales and conditions, and even conditions in familiar locales, can vary greatly. A precaution you can take to avoid stress is to know your diving limits and stay within them. Diving in unfamiliar conditions or in situations beyond your skill level can lead to stress.

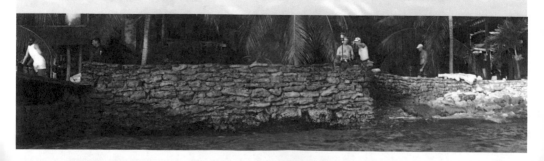

In diving it is never a good idea to show off, or succumb to peer pressure because you fear social embarrassment. If you are uncomfortable with the conditions, choose not to dive, or change your diving location.

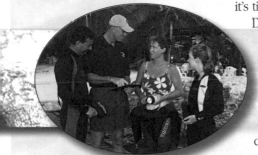

If you want to improve or expand your abilities, it's time for specialty training. Night, Wreck, and Deep Diving are potentially dangerous for the untrained diver. You may have logged a hundred dives in the deep, cold waters of Lake Michigan exploring wrecks, but that does not qualify you for diving in the kelp beds of California. Whenever encountering unfamiliar conditions, safe divers will either dive with someone trained in that type of diving, get special training, or refrain from diving. Local dive stores offer specialty training for their local conditions, as well as charter and group dives.

In unfamiliar conditions, dive with someone trained in that type of diving.

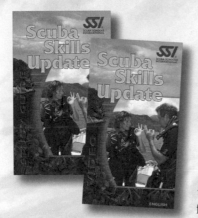

An annual Scuba Skills Update will boost your confidence.

Lack of Skills and Training

Stress can be caused by lack of skill, lack of specialty training, lack of practice, or failure to update skills annually. Many divers need but don't get an annual update, and therefore may be out of practice when going diving for the first time after a lengthy break. This lack of skill could translate into moving at a slower pace, having difficulty with equipment, or forgetting basic routines. For example, a diver who is already fatigued at the end of a dive often forgets to power inflate his/her BC upon surfacing. This in turn leads to the need to tread water, further increasing fatigue and stress. Being out of step like this can cause a feeling of insecurity and under confidence, which can be stressful. An annual Scuba Skills Update and occasional practice will boost your confidence in your abilities. Consult with your SSI Dive Center about enrolling in an SSI Scuba Skills Update program if your skills need refreshing.

Lack of skill is most stressful during an emergency situation. You may know a skill, but forget how to perform it when necessary. Properly learned skills are nothing more than conditioned responses. The conditioning will diminish with lack of use, and maintaining a high skill level requires repetition.

A solid grasp of basic diving skills can turn physically weaker or mentally anxious individuals into safer divers than their stronger counterparts. Also, being able to perform self-aid and buddy-assist skills competently, and being comfortable with your equipment are two key steps to avoiding stress when diving. However, learning your scuba skills is not enough; they must be repeatedly practiced and rehearsed in order for you to stay finely tuned.

Overlearning of Skills

All the basic scuba skills should be overlearned until they become automatic responses, especially the self-aid and emergency skills. Many skills are used every time you dive, but others, such as rescue procedures, are used only in an emergency situation. These skills are the most critical for survival yet they are the easiest forgotten because they may never be performed again after you finish your certification course. This is why practice and rehearsal are so important.

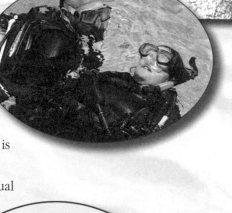

Practice can come in more forms than actual physical rehearsal, it can also come in the form of mental rehearsal (imagery), or visual rehearsal; a combination of these forms of practice will be the most beneficial. Physical rehearsal includes getting into the pool or open water on occasion to practice your scuba skills. You may not have the opportunity to go on a dive trip more than once a year, but that does not mean you can't go to the local pool or lake for some practice.

Scuba Skills Update

If you only dive once a year, it is also recommended to get an annual Scuba Skills Update from your local dive store. An Update allows you the chance to practice under supervision of an instructor, break bad habits, and catch up on new skills and pieces of equipment.

DIVER DIAMOND *SSI*
KNOWLEDGE · SKILLS · EQUIPMENT · EXPERIENCE

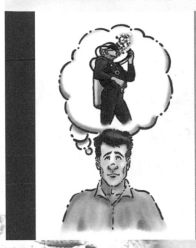

Mental Rehearsal

Mental imagery is a valuable tool that can be performed anytime, anywhere. Part of your pre-dive preparation should include mentally rehearsing the events of the upcoming dive. Actually imagine yourself gearing up, entering the water, descending and feeling yourself equalize your ears. Imagine what you will be doing throughout the dive and how you will handle yourself. When it is time to ascend, think about the procedure, relax, and imagine yourself as you swim towards the surface. This practice will help to relax you and will keep you practiced in the skills needed for diving.

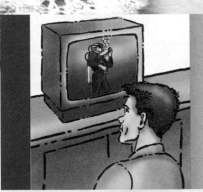

Visual Rehearsal

People also learn visually by observation. You may want to sit in on a dive class, watch a TV show on diving, or watch a video tape on scuba skills such as the SSI Open Water Diver DVD or the SSI Scuba Skills Update DVD. The visual reminder can help refresh your memory and keep you mentally in-tune with your diving skills.

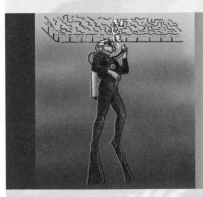

Physical Rehearsal

Practice all of your skills, especially those you have difficulty performing efficiently. Practice will build mental confidence and perfect your physical talents. Emergency procedures should be practiced with these three methods whenever possible. The more automatic these skills become, the safer diving will be for you and your buddy.

Proper Weight and Buoyancy Control

Proper weighting and buoyancy control is one of the most important skills for diving comfort. If you can easily maintain neutral buoyancy at any depth, you have made a great stride towards eliminating stress. If you are negatively buoyant and must fight to stay off the bottom, or conversely, too buoyant and can't keep from floating, you may be "on edge" and distracted. The need to continually adjust your buoyancy will keep your mind preoccupied, taking it away from the pleasures of the diving experience.

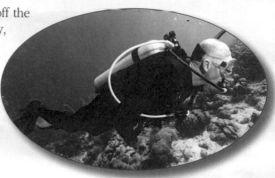

The ability to stay neutrally buoyant will help prevent stress.

Some divers will slightly overweight themselves on purpose to facilitate getting below the surface more easily. Others overweight themselves by accident; they appear to need more weight only because they cannot completely relax under water. Divers that are not relaxed will not fully exhale all the air from their lungs so this will keep them positively buoyant, thus appearing that they need more weight. This situation is dangerous because an overweighted diver at the surface will continue to become heavier during descent. In contrast, when an overweighted diver begins to surface, their rate of ascent will accelerate as they reach the surface because of all the air in their BC that was necessary to compensate for the extra weight on their belt. Another factor is the positive buoyancy created by an empty cylinder at the end of a dive.

80 CF Aluminum Cylinder Buoyancy

Full = -3 to -5 lbs
(-1.36 to -2.27 kg.)

Empty = +2 to +4 lbs.
(+.9 to +1.8 kg.)

Most aluminium 80 CF cylinders have 2 to 5 pounds/.9 to 2.27 kilograms of positive buoyancy when close to empty. This added buoyancy will increase your rate of ascent as you near 30 feet/10 metres, and make safety stops at 15 feet/5 metres more challenging.

If you normally breathe your cylinder to the 500 psi/35 bar minimum recommended air pressure, you may want to add an additional 1 to 3 pounds/.5 to 1.36 kilograms of weight (after establishing your proper weighting at the surface) to compensate for this extra positive buoyancy.

However, if you end each dive with around 1000 psi/70 bar you will not have to worry about the positive buoyancy of your cylinder. True neutral buoyancy should be established at the surface, and you should be able to float at eye level with no air in your BC or lungs. If you are truly neutrally buoyant, getting below the surface can be difficult and may require the use of a line to pull yourself down, or an upward sweeping of your arms. Once you are at 15 feet/5 metres, descending will be easy. Neutral buoyancy should be able to be maintained under water with only a small inflation or deflation of the vest, or inhalation and exhalation of your lungs.

A perfectly weighted diver will require only small buoyancy adjustments of the BC when diving.

Every buoyancy compensator and power inflator works differently. If you are using a new BC, familiarize yourself with the location of controls, and with its buoyancy characteristics, for example, how much inflation it takes to get you to neutral buoyancy at depth.

Alternate Air Source Breathing

Various types of alternate air systems are available, and each works differently. Some are attached to the BC inflator hose on the left side of the jacket, others are independent of the Air Delivery System. Become familiar with different configurations and how they operate, and keep up with the changes in the equipment market. Visit your local SSI Dive Center and ask for a demonstration of various types of alternate air sources. This knowledge will prepare you for an air emergency. Also be sure to familiarize yourself with your buddy's Total Diving System during the pre-dive buddy check.

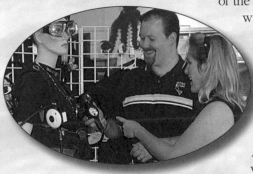

Your local dive store can provide information on equipment.

Emergency Ascents and Weight Ditching

First of all, secure your weight the same way every time. If you are using a weight belt, the buckle is located front and centre and the release always opens the same way with your strong hand. As you progress through the dive, check the positioning of the weight occasionally and readjust it, and make sure other equipment is not interfering with easy access to the release mechanism.

Alternate Air Source Rehearsal

Use mental imaging to rehearse alternate air source breathing. Rehearse the skill, as the donor and needer alternately. Imagine yourself controlling your buddy's panic as you offer an air source and make reassuring physical contact. Imagine the loss of your air, and imagine remaining in control as you signal your buddy for help.

KNOWLEDGE • SKILLS • DIVER DIAMOND • SSI • EQUIPMENT • EXPERIENCE

Each time you dive you should mentally rehearse emergency ascent procedures.

The best place to practice an emergency ascent is on every normal ascent you make. Mentally rehearse the steps that would be taken should it be necessary to make an emergency ascent. Locate the belt and buckle, and mentally drop it. Then practice flaring your body in the last 20 feet/6 metres, reducing the risk of embolism, assuring yourself that you will be at the surface and breathing freely within seconds. And, of course, practice exhaling continuously during your ascent, or attempting to breathe from the second-stage regulator, keeping your airway open despite a loss of air.

The reason for preparation is, naturally, to prevent the kind of stress that can lead to accidents. You have just learned a few things about preventing stress through knowledge, experience, practice — both mental and actual — proper maintenance and updating of equipment, fitness, and first aid. True preparedness does not assume that stress will never occur, but knowing you are prepared will increase your confidence in yourself and your dive plan.

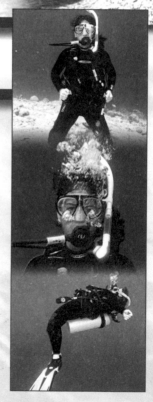

Mentally rehearse emergency procedures on every ascent.

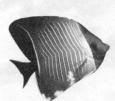

Summary

You shouldn't assume that diver stress will inevitably show up at some time during your years as a scuba diver. Knowing the causes, in fact, is the first step in learning exactly how to avoid them and consequently prevent stress from occurring. It is quite possible to dive comfortably and enjoyably throughout your experience as a diver. However, knowing the causes of stress can help you detect stress in your buddy or fellow diving companions. True preparedness is knowing what to do when stress occurs while diving.

You can never know what your panic threshold is until you are put to the test — several stressors suddenly combining to cause you difficulty which must be dealt with immediately. You must also be prepared — as in the defensive diver — to "watch out for the other guy."

In the next section we will look at the behavioral signs you can use to detect stress, and how to deal with stress should it arise.

2

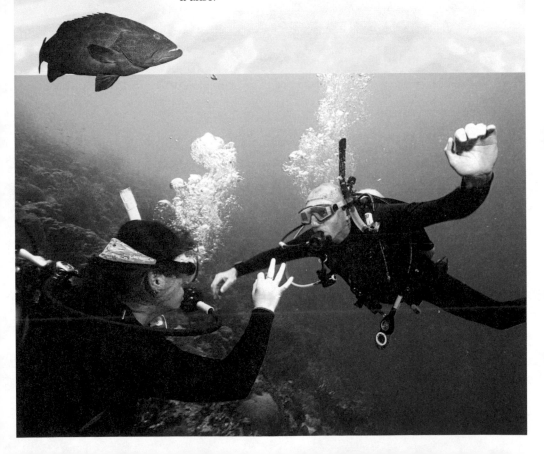

Section 2 Review Questions

1. Stress usually originates in divers because: (List five reasons)

   _____

   _____

   _____

   _____

   _____

2

2. An unfit person may also have a hard time _____ or
   _____ a buddy in need.

3. Monitor yourself and buddy for _____ throughout the
   day, being ready to abort before _____ strikes.

4. By definition, water below _____ is considered cold,
   due to the fact that body heat is absorbed _____ times
   faster in water than air.

5. Psychological contraindications to diving include: (List two)

   _____

   _____

6. If your buddy seems nervous or anxious, constant
   _____ through hand signals,
   _____ , _____ , and
   _____ _____ will provide
   encouragement.

7. Always stay within sight of each other, and if visibility is low,
   establish _____ _____ such
   as _____ _____ .

8. Since it is a much more common problem than running out of air,
   _____ _____ may be the
   single largest contributor to stress.

9. When diving in either extremely _____ or
_____ water it is hard to estimate
_____ visually.

10. Being well-trained, well-equipped, and even highly experienced
does not necessarily qualify a diver as "_____ ."

11. Whenever necessary, _____ ,
_____ , or _____ a dive that
involves potentially hazardous environmental conditions.

12. Diving in _____ _____
or in situations beyond your _____
_____ can lead to stress.

13. Properly learned skills are nothing more than
_____ _____ .

14. Practice can come in more forms than actual physical rehearsal,
it can also come in the form of _____
_____ (imagery), or _____
_____ ; a combination of these forms of
practice will be most beneficial .

15. The reason for _____ is, naturally, to
prevent the kind of _____ that can lead to
_____ .

Detecting & Dealing with Stress

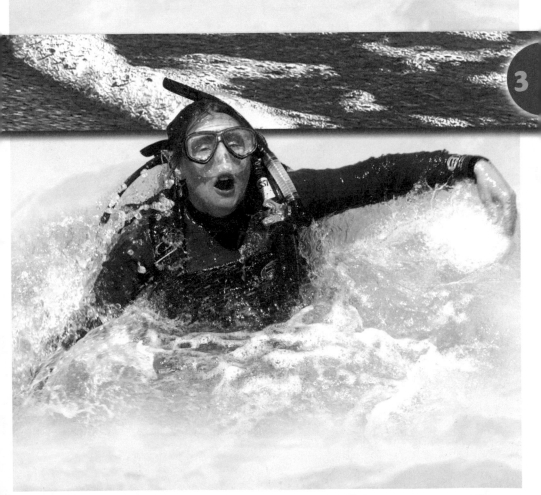

here are certain behavioral signs that signal when stress
is present in your buddy; and if you're paying attention,
in yourself. These signs can occur in one of three stages:
Stage 1: Before the Dive, Stage 2: During the Dive, and
Stage 3: End of the Dive.

Section 3 Objectives
After completing this section you will be able to:

◆ List the signs of stress during the three stages
   of a dive,

◆ Understand how to avoid and manage
   stress during the three stages of a dive.

Early detection of stress in any stage is
advantageous, but Stage 1 is probably the most
important time to treat problems that might otherwise
lead to stress in Stage 2, when the dive is already underway.

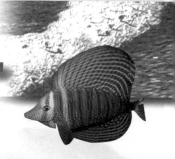

If stress is detected and dealt with immediately, the dive
may continue as planned. The further along stress is allowed
to progress, the more difficult the situation becomes, and the
more likely panic and accident will result. When you detect
stress in your buddy, you need to immediately assess the
source of that stress and deal with it appropriately. Proper
identification is as important as early detection. An inaccurate
solution may be better than none at all, but it may not be
good enough to prevent stress from leading to panic.

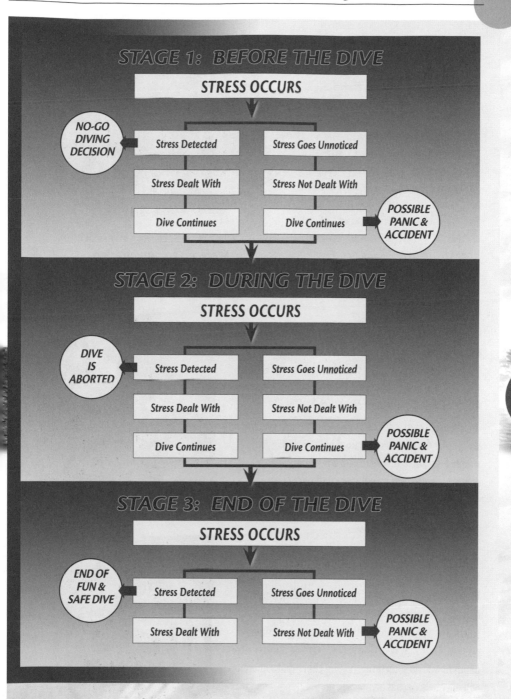

Stage 1: Before the Dive

The key to detecting stress in Stage 1 is communication. In the pre-dive phase, communication between you and your buddy is much easier than it is under water. You are able to detect subtleties in your buddy's behavior that wouldn't be as apparent in the water. Communicate your own unresolved problems — such as uncertainty about a dive plan — to avoid stress personally, but also be very attentive to your buddy. A certain amount of nervous anticipation before a dive is to be expected, but abnormal behaviors should warrant concern.

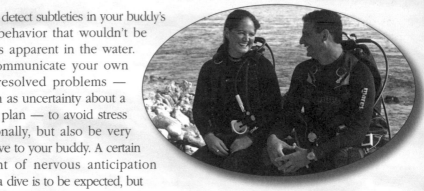

The key to detecting stress in Stage 1 is communication

Preoccupation

Divers who are preoccupied may not pay attention to you as you try to speak to them. If your buddy seems distant while you are making your dive plan, for example, he or she may be trying to block out external stressors, such as worrying that the weather might turn bad.

Another sign of preoccupation is forgetfulness, which is a sign that the person is not thinking clearly. Forgetting simple tasks such as hooking up a power inflator or securing weight may signal stress or discomfort.

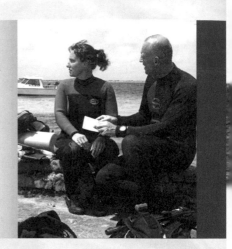

Difficulty with Equipment

If buddies have difficulty with, or delay assembling, adjusting, locating, or putting on equipment, it could be a sign of stress, especially if they are making unfounded excuses. They may be trying to cover up any uncertainty about how to do something, hoping either that someone will offer help or that no one will notice. It may be that they are having trouble with a normally simple task because of tension or preoccupation.

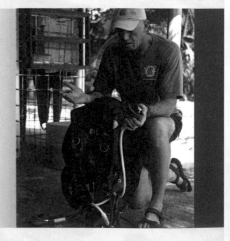

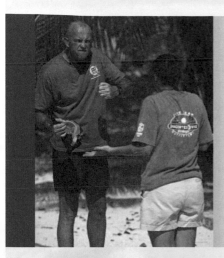

Irritability and Frustration

While some laugh about possible danger, others grow short-tempered. They may snap, criticize, or lose patience for little or no reason. Since a dive trip is a social and recreational activity, there is normally no reason to be irritable.

Frustration caused by an inability to perform to one's own standard is another sign of stress. Frustrated people may become abusive to others, or complicate matters for themselves by adding their emotions to an existing stressor.

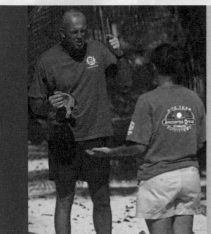

Superiority

Some people try to make others feel inferior in order to bolster their own sense of superiority. This behavior is usually masking a lack of confidence, or a fear of incompetence. They may be trying to convince themselves and others that they are completely in control — a way of falsely building the confidence that they may lack. Beware of those who act superior, because they may actually lack the knowledge, training, and experience they try to convey. Truly confident people don't feel the need to flaunt their knowledge.

3

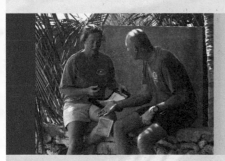

Other Changes in Behavior

Silence, hyperactivity, humor, seriousness, tardiness, and clumsiness are but a few signs of possible stress. These behaviors could be signaling common nervousness, but when buddies behave in ways alien to their nature, there is probably something wrong.

Dealing with Stress in Stage 1

A safe dive starts with pre-dive planning. This includes making a dive plan that both buddies are comfortable with, and also

making sure both buddies are comfortable with their
equipment and with each other before entering the water.
Pre-dive stress can be caused by something as simple as
going to a new dive site, diving with a new buddy, or making
the first dive of the trip. Just by making sure you and your
buddy are both comfortable, you may be eliminating stress
from your entire dive.

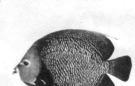

Make a Good Dive Plan

A good dive plan is critical because it can eliminate fear of
the unknown by answering questions up front. If both buddies
understand the plan, and understand contingencies such as a
lost buddy procedure, both will be more comfortable going
into the dive. There are several elements of a good dive plan:

Discuss the Objective of the Dive

Both buddies must agree on the objective of the dive,
whether it is taking photos or exploring a wreck. Diving
for different purposes can encourage splitting
up. If you agree on one objective, you will
both know what to expect, and you'll be in
"sync" mentally as well as physically. Special
equipment may also be needed for certain
dive objectives, such as deep diving, and if
this is not planned for, you both may get
caught in a situation for which you are
not prepared.

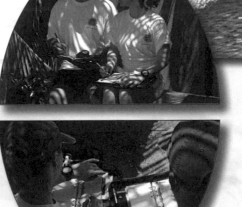

Set Parameters to which Both Buddies Agree

After agreeing on a purpose, set your
parameters. Agree on depth, bottom time,
compass headings, physical parameters
of the dive (for instance, diving along
a coral wall and returning when you
reach a certain landmark), and minimum
psi/bar remaining in your cylinder before
you begin a return to an entry point. Most
importantly, after setting parameters, stick to
them. If you stray from the parameters, your buddy
may become anxious or frightened. Also, when planning
no-decompression dives, use your computer or dive tables
conservatively and add the extra assurance of always making
a three to five minute stop at 15 feet/5 metres. A sure cause of

Computers

Each diver must dive with their own computer. Do not depend on your buddy's computer for your safety. Each diver will have slight variances in their dive plan that will affect their diving profile, especially during an entire week of diving.

worry is uncertainty about whether or not you'll have to make a decompression stop.

Part of being conservative with depths and times includes using computers intelligently on repetitive dives, and multi-level, multi-day diving. It is unwise to dive all week and still expect total safety from a dive computer. Personal factors such as fatigue, dehydration, alcohol, and body fat content give each diver a different level of susceptibility to decompression sickness. Plan a rest day during resort and charter trips, usually on the third or fourth day, and always make a decompression stop for three to five minutes at 15 feet/5 metres on every dive.

Discuss Training Methods

Your training in emergency skills such as alternate air source breathing may vary from your buddy's training.

Before your dive, discuss how each of you performs emergency skills (or precautionary skills such as a safety stop before surfacing) and agree on similar methods.

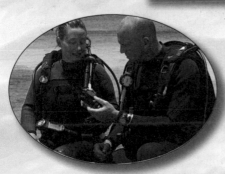

Unless discussed, when it comes time to perform emergency skills you may not be able to coordinate with your buddy.

Hand signals should also be decided on before diving. Some divers do not utilize all the signals, and others develop their own. Agreement on signals will decrease the chance of stress from unintelligible communication and increase your ability to exchange information and share the diving experience.

Discuss emergency procedures before diving

Discuss How Equipment Functions

It is possible that you or your buddy have a piece of equipment with which the other is not familiar. BCs and weight systems come with different buckle mechanisms, and power inflator systems vary by manufacturer. There are also a variety of alternate air source configurations available. Be sure you know how each other's equipment functions so that you can assist in an emergency.

Plan for Possible Problems or Changes

It is important to be flexible, and to be willing to alter your plans to meet the demands of the dive. For instance, if you had planned to dive a wreck, but once you reached it you saw an eagle ray nearby and wanted to descend to get a closer look, you would need to alter your original planned depth. This is why it is a good idea in such a case to always dive with a computer or have your dive table with you, possibly kept in a pocket of your BC, in case you are not diving with a computer. You will need to communicate with your buddy

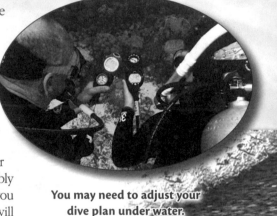

You may need to adjust your dive plan under water.

and both agree to make the change in your plan, then figure a new bottom time if necessary. Planning ahead for such a scenario, you may want to allow a margin in your plan so that you can stay longer or go deeper if you so desire.

Also plan how to deal with specific problems that could occur. For example, if you're diving in an area which is known to have a strong current, plan your entry and exit points and your route of travel such that you avoid it, and also discuss exactly what you'll do if by chance you get caught in the current.

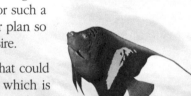

Create a Positive Environment Through Communication and Support

Buddies must feel confident in each other's abilities, and in each other's presence. A poor buddy may try to make a partner feel intimidated or inferior by boasting about knowledge and experience, or may try to pressure a buddy

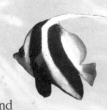

to conform to a rigorous dive plan or to dive beyond his or her limits. These are all negative situations which can cause stress.

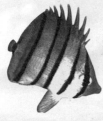

A good buddy will create a sense of trust and ease through communication, encouragement, support, and respect. If you feel you can depend on your buddy, you can relax and enjoy the dive. If you are open and honest with each other, you will be more likely to detect signs of stress. That is, if you know each other's equipment and have made a dive plan that fits both of your ability levels, you will probably notice if your partner is suddenly displaying abnormal behavior. Also, get used to helping each other on land so that helping each other under water will come naturally.

Discuss the Go, No-Go Diving Decision

A major source of stress is feeling that you must go ahead with a dive when you know you aren't able to or do not wish to. Divers may feel pressured to go along with the group even when they feel sick, fatigued, or are lacking a piece of equipment. Instead, divers should get used to the idea that it's okay to back out if necessary, without fear of embarrassment. Such reassurance may at times be all that is needed to calm whatever anxieties they are having so that they can go ahead with the dive.

Take time to weigh all the factors when deciding when to go, or not to go.

Factors that justify a no-go diving decision include:

♦ Poor environmental conditions,

♦ Equipment problems,

♦ Missing equipment,

♦ Improper training for the conditions, and

♦ Sickness.

Keep an eye on conditions, and thoroughly check your equipment.

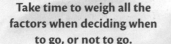

If anything out-of-the-ordinary happens in the planning phase, reassess your dive decision. Remember, there is always another vacation or diving day. Don't pressure yourself just because you have traveled a great distance. Your health and safety is always top priority!

Do a Pre-Entry Buddy Check

Once you and your buddy are geared up, you should make a last minute check of your equipment and your dive plan. Make sure your hoses are not tangled and that the weight release mechanism is accessible. Confirm that your air supplies are turned on, and that both primary and alternate air sources are working properly. You should also quickly review hand signals and your dive parameters. If your dive decision is still a "go," then it is time to enter. The last minute check can prevent stress and build confidence by confirming your comfort with your equipment, dive plan, and dive decision.

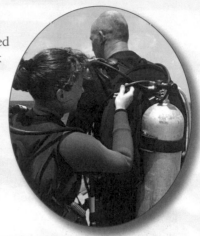

A pre-entry check can build confidence and prevent stress.

Stage 2: During the Dive

If neither you nor your buddy are experiencing pre-dive stress, the dive will go on as planned. But as you begin the dive there are still many situations that can trigger stress. Many times stress may not even occur until you actually enter the water. For example, the water may be extremely cold, your mask may dislodge, or you may make a clumsy entry and become disoriented.

If stress does occur during the dive, it can still be dealt with. Again, the earlier it is detected, the better your chances of continuing the dive. Stress is more dangerous under water, so behavior should be watched more carefully. The further stress builds, the more conspicuous behavior will become. Be alert for signs of stress and remember, it is not the presence of one sign, but the combination of signs that should warrant concern.

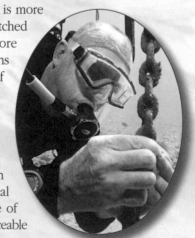

Contact Maintenance

Contact maintenance is a term used to describe the stress response in which an individual intensely tries to maintain physical (and psychological) contact with a source of security.[1] This behavior will probably be noticeable

---

[1]Arthur Bachrach & Glen Egstrom, *Stress and Performance in Diving* (San Pedro: Best, 1987, p. 18

at the beginning of the dive. Your buddy may not want to let go of the boat, ladder, anchor line, or you. If this behavior is present, encourage your buddy to surface so you can discuss the problem.

Once your point of descent is reached and the dive is about to begin, stress may appear in the form of second thoughts, delays, and nervousness. Excessive ear clearing and last minute gear adjustments may be forms of stalling and signs of psychological discomfort. If this stress goes unnoticed and is not dealt with, it will likely increase.

If your buddy feels apprehensive, allow him or her to abort the dive. Don't force him or her to proceed under stress.

Breathing and Air Supply

Since a diver's air supply is crucial for survival, problems with breathing under water can be a source of great stress. Many things can affect breathing resistance in addition to stress such as:

◆ Cold water,

◆ A restrictive wet suit,

◆ Depth,

◆ Low cylinder pressure, and

◆ Poor equipment maintenance.

Breathing resistance can cause rapid, shallow breathing, and this can lead to an imbalance in the gases of the respiratory system (as described by the psycho-respiratory cycle in Section 1).

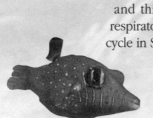

A sign of rapid, shallow breathing is an almost continuous exhalation of a large amount of bubbles. Normal breathing should appear as a slow, steady inhalation followed by a slow, steady exhalation.

Buoyancy Control

Persons under stress will have increased muscle tension and problems relaxing, so their movements may appear rigid and jerky. This failure to relax will cause buoyancy control problems because the diver will feel overweighted and will overcompensate by continuously adding air to the BC. The diver may even feel the need to continuously swim or use their arms and legs in an effort to control his or her buoyancy.

Poor buoyancy control can signal stress.

Proper buoyancy control begins with proper weighting and continues with relaxation and proper breathing. It is a continuous cycle in that stress causes problems with buoyancy control, while buoyancy problems lead to stress.

Excessive Behavior

Excessive behavior such as the repeated checking and adjusting can signal stress. This could be caused by discomfort. An unwillingness to let go of the power inflator, for example, could indicate fear of a loss of buoyancy control. A repeated tugging at the wet suit could signal a painful pressure spot. Both types of behavior can signal stress.

RAPID BREATHING & FAILURE TO RELAX

CONTINUOUS USE OF ARMS & LEGS OR DUMPING AIR FROM BC.

OVERWEIGHTED OR FEELING OF BEING OVERWEIGHTED

RAPID BREATHING & FAILURE TO RELAX

Buoyancy/stress cycle.

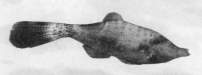
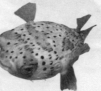

Inability to Communicate

General stress or the sudden occurrence or appearance of a stressor might result in a wide-eyed expression. Monitor your buddy for the wide-eyed look and for any fixation of vision.

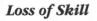

If your fellow diver is unable to recognize you or react to your presence, beware; severe stress may be present and panic could result.

Wide-eyed expression

A buddy's inability to respond or communicate may not include the wide-eyed expression however. Your buddy may try to block out all outside stressors and consequently become introverted. This trance-like state may be broken by your attempts to communicate, but if there is no response to hand signals or physical contact, stress is present and well on the way to becoming panic.

Loss of Skill

A diver experiencing stress may become mentally engrossed in their situation and forget how to perform basic skills. Although your buddy has been trained in how to switch from one second-stage regulator to another, stress caused by the failure of the primary air source may cause a lack of coordination, fear, confusion, or even an absolute inability to perform. Stress which is already present may also lead to a loss of skill. If you are preoccupied with getting to the surface because you are running low on air, you may forget that weight ditching is the best way to get to the surface and stay there. The failure to perform can then compound the stress and result in panic and/or an accident.

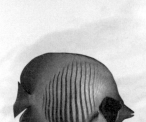

Dealing with Stress in Stage 2

Knowing how to respond to stress as the dive gets under way might make the difference in the dive continuing, and it could be the point at which small problems can be taken care of so that they don't develop into much more difficult situations. There are several ways to deal with stress as divers enter the water, and after the dive has begun.

Use the Easiest Methods of Entry and Descent

Never complicate the entry process and chance difficulty; always use the safest, easiest method of entry for prevailing conditions. If you do not know which entry to use, ask a local diver or a local dive store. When diving from a boat, the boat captain or dive master will explain which method to use. No matter what kind of entry you use, always cover your mask and second-stage regulator with one hand so that they aren't lost on entry, and have enough air in your BC to allow you to float.

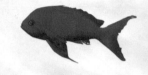

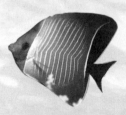

A descent line provides a good reference point.

Once in the water, use the easiest method of descent, too. Descending in a feet down, head up position will usually make it easier to equalize your ears and control your rate of descent. Begin to equalize before descending, then equalize continually as you go deeper, ascending a few feet if necessary to relieve any discomfort you may feel.

You should have a visual reference point for your descent so that you can easily find the same place when you're ready to ascend. In poor visibility, be sure and take a compass heading. A descent line provides a good reference point, and it also provides for a more controllable descent because it allows you to hang on and move downward at your own pace instead of free-floating in water.

Good buoyancy control is another important skill for safe descents. Controlling your buoyancy as you descend means setting your own pace, and it means the ability to stabilize at a planned depth from which you'll start your exploration. It is important to stop and relax for a few moments once you have reached your planned depth so that you can get

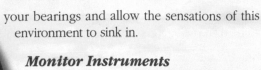

your bearings and allow the sensations of this environment to sink in.

Monitor Instruments

During a dive you must monitor how much air you have remaining so you can plan your return trip when necessary, and you must monitor depth and time to make sure you're staying within your no-decompression limits.

Be Aware of Physical Stress and Monitor Limitations

If you are cautious with your own physical and mental limits, stress should not develop. Throughout your dive occasionally stop, rest, and evaluate your physical condition. Are you tired, or cold? Breathing harder than normal? Using more air than normal? All of these signs can indicate the onset of fatigue. If you do not feel recuperated after your rest, it is time to end the dive.

3

Never feel the need to rush when diving, but move in a slow, relaxed manner. When diving with a group, move at the pace of the slowest buddy to help them from becoming fatigued.

Keep in Constant Contact With Your Buddy

Communicate with your buddy not only through hand signals, but also through physical contact and eye contact. Also swim side-by-side instead of in a line so that you can easily maintain contact and communication.

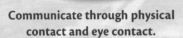

Communicate through physical contact and eye contact.

Let buddies know that you are there, that you care, and that you are paying attention to them. Share the experience with them. Reassurance from a buddy can prevent stress.

One of the most important things to monitor is breathing pattern. If your own breathing becomes rapid and shallow, stop and think about what is bothering you and what you need to do to regain control. If your buddy is breathing irregularly, bring his or her attention to it so that the cause can be discerned and breathing can be returned to normal.

If you are alert and observant, you should easily be able to detect stress in either yourself or your buddy. If you are prepared with a high level of fitness, a proper Total Diving System, and a good dive plan, you should be able to deal with any stressful situation that may arise. Mental strength and preparedness can prevent a simple self-aid situation from turning into a buddy assist or buddy rescue.

Stage 3: End of the Dive

Even after successfully completing a dive, divers are not immune to stress. The final ascent and surface swim can involve stress producing problems. In fact, stress at the end of a dive is common due to fatigue and low cylinder pressure. It is possible to lose direction, which would require an extended return trip to an exit point or a long swim against a current or surface chop.

Surface procedures are the most poorly performed in diving. A significant number of divers have drowned on the surface by failing to inflate their BCs or drop their weight belts when necessary. In over 90% of diving fatalities, the victim failed to drop the weight.[2] Watch your buddy closely for proper performance of surface procedures. He or she should be stable and relaxed.

Contrary to the stereotypical image, the drowning victim usually does not scream for help and wave energetically on the surface, but rather drops silently below the surface unseen and unheard.

Remember that the dive is not over until both buddies are safely on the shore or boat. Be aware of the following signs of stress at the end of your dive.

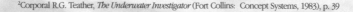

[2]Corporal R.G. Teather, *The Underwater Investigator* (Fort Collins: Concept Systems, 1983), p. 39

Failure to Achieve Positive Buoyancy

A diver who fails to achieve positive buoyancy on the surface will be forced to tread water to stay afloat. If you observe your buddy struggling at the surface, chances are the simple skill of BC inflation has been forgotten due to other stress factors.

Mask off, Regulator Removed

Often, a stressed or panicked diver will quickly remove the mask and/ or second-stage regulator when surfacing. Because stress creates real or imagined breathing difficulty, an attempt is being made to breathe freely. Breathing straight from the mouth and nose seems logical; however, if environmental conditions are poor, if the diver's face has not quite reached the surface, or if there is failure to achieve positive buoyancy, the diver may breathe water and become a candidate for drowning.

Shortness of Breath

When breathing is rapid and shallow under water it will usually continue to be shallow on the surface, and until you relax, it will be difficult to inhale a full lung of air. As long as breathing remains shallow you will feel deprived of oxygen, so stress will continue. Once on the surface, continue to monitor your own and your buddy's breathing, and make necessary adjustments to your equipment and exposure suit for less restriction.

Signs of Drowning

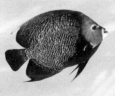

Most people fail to recognize the signs of drowning. The image of the alert lifeguard who saves the day by tossing a ring buoy to a grateful victim is pure fiction. This might work for a strong swimmer who is fatigued, but not a true drowning victim. A person who is drowning is in a state of panic, totally consumed by the need to breathe and stay above water; there is an inability to see, hear, react to instructions, or call out for help.

All buddies should be able to recognize the following three signs of drowning:

1. **Head Held Back and Out of Water.**

The victim's main objective is to keep the head above water at all costs. Drowning victims know instinctively that if their heads go below the surface they will inhale more water. Holding the head back is another instinctive reaction which opens the airway and gets the mouth as high as possible above water.

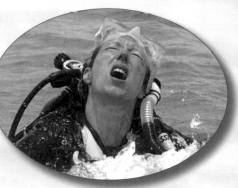

Head held back and out of water.

2. **Arms Attempting to Push Out the Water.**

The slapping arm movement of a drowning victim is an instinctive attempt to keep the head above water. Unlike the waving arms we think of in a non-panic victim, the drowning victim pushes downward, with both arms partially extended from the sides.

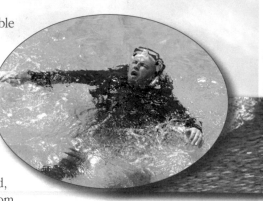

Arms attempting to push out of the water.

3. **Inability to Speak.**

Both breathing and speech are functions of the respiratory system, but when drowning, speech is overruled by the primary need to breathe.[3] This means the victim will be unable to call for help.

Dealing with Stress in Stage 3

At the end of the dive you may be cold, tired, and low on air — a prime candidate for stress and an accident. Intelligent ascent and surface procedures can help you prevent stress at the end of the dive.

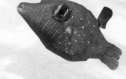

Plan to End your Dive with 500 psi/35 bar

A well planned return trip may prevent many problems at the end of the dive. By using a compass and visual points of reference, you can quickly return as near to your exit point

[3] Frank Pia, "Observationas of Drowning of Non-Swimmers." *The Journal of Physical Education.* July/Aug. 1978, pp. 164-181

as possible. Predetermine the time you'll need to return, and estimate the required air supply. Allow a margin of safety by planning to end the dive following a safety stop at 15 feet/5 metres, with no less than 500 psi/35 bar; **do not wait** until you have 500 psi/35 bar left before you begin your ascent, or you may find yourself low on air and unable to find your exit point.

Control Your Ascents

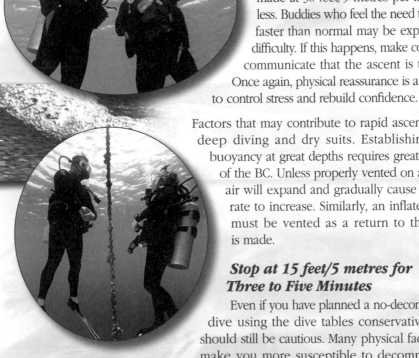

The overwhelming desire to reach the surface, whether because of the need for air or from other causes, should be avoided. All normal ascents should be made at 30 feet/9 metres per minute or less. Buddies who feel the need to surface faster than normal may be experiencing difficulty. If this happens, make contact and communicate that the ascent is too rapid. Once again, physical reassurance is a good way to control stress and rebuild confidence.

Factors that may contribute to rapid ascents include deep diving and dry suits. Establishing neutral buoyancy at great depths requires greater inflation of the BC. Unless properly vented on ascent, this air will expand and gradually cause the ascent rate to increase. Similarly, an inflated dry suit must be vented as a return to the surface is made.

Stop at 15 feet/5 metres for Three to Five Minutes

Even if you have planned a no-decompression dive using the dive tables conservatively, you should still be cautious. Many physical factors can make you more susceptible to decompression sickness, including age, dehydration, body weight, level of fitness, and excess nitrogen absorption due to repeated dives on successive days. So, for an extra margin of safety, always make a safety stop on every dive.

Make a safety stop on every dive.

Ditch Any Equipment that is Creating Drag

As you make your return trip, ascent, or surface swim to your exit point, be aware of your level of physical exertion.

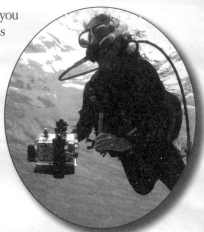

Take rest breaks when necessary, but if you become fatigued and a rest break does not help, you may need to ditch any hand-held equipment that is creating a drag. It is possible that a buddy might be able to carry the equipment for you, though it is more likely that he or she, too, would be nearing energy limits. Camera equipment, goody bags, fish stringers, and spear guns all create drag (and they can always be retrieved later). It is more desirable to lose equipment than it is to risk overexertion, panic, or a heart attack.

Become Positively Buoyant on the Surface

When you reach the surface, immediately become positively buoyant.

You may need to ditch any hand-held equipment that is creating a drag.

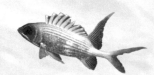

Surface buoyancy allows you to keep your head above water and rest comfortably without having to tread water.

If you need to swim to your exit point, take a few moments to rest at the surface by using your BC to suspend you in water. Gaining buoyancy at the surface should be an automatic skill; a contingency skill for additional buoyancy at the surface is weight ditching.

Use the Easiest Method of Swimming and Breathing at the Surface

When swimming on the surface, take slow, easy kicks in a face-down position, and swim on your back for brief periods as an alternative. Adjust the buoyancy of the BC so that it doesn't uncomfortably restrict breathing or create excess drag. Use your snorkel to breathe through, or continue to use the second-stage regulator — especially if there is surface chop or you are moving through breaking water.

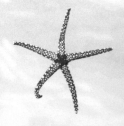

Use the Easiest Method of Exit

As when entering the water, use the easiest method of exit for your situation. Before ever entering the water you should do a pre-dive scouting of an exit point. This exit point should be one that can easily be found after surfacing, should not be in an area of heavy water action or rocky shoreline, and should not be heading against the direction of a current. When boat diving, the captain or dive master will inform you of how to exit.

If you are not sure of how or where to exit in a dive location, ask a local SSI Dive Center, or ask experienced divers in the area.

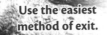
Use the easiest method of exit.

No matter what type of exit you use, always exit with some air in your BC, and your mask and second-stage regulator (or snorkel) in place. This insures that you will be able to see, breathe, and float until you are safely out of the water.

Summary

In learning how to detect and deal with stress we begin to express the real importance of our role as a safe diver and a good, reliable buddy. As you learn more about diver stress and how to notice its causes and its onset, you are further enabling yourself to reduce or eliminate it.

In the next section we will examine accident management and what to do should stress progress into an accident situation.

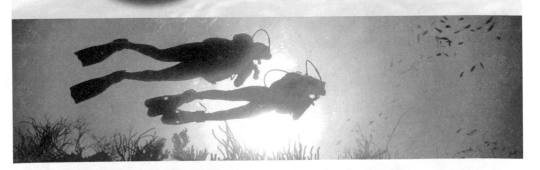

Section 3 Review Questions

1. The further along stress is allowed to progress, the more difficult the situation becomes, and the more likely _____ and _____ will result.

2. Another sign of _____ is _____ , which is a sign that the person is not thinking clearly.

3. _____ caused by an inability to perform to one's own standard is another sign of _____ .

4. _____ , _____ , _____ , _____ , _____ , and _____ are but a few signs of possible stress.

5. Pre-dive stress can be caused by something as simple as going to a new _____ _____ , diving with a _____ _____ , or making the _____ _____ of the trip.

6. Part of being conservative with depths and times includes using computers intelligently on _____ dives, and _____ , _____ diving.

7. A good buddy will create a sense of trust and ease through _____ , _____ , _____ , and _____ .

8. Divers should get used to the idea that it's okay to back out if necessary, without fear of _____ .

9. Once your point of descent is reached and the dive is about to begin, stress may appear in the form of _____ _____ , _____ , and _____ .

10. Persons under stress will have increased muscle tension and problems relaxing, so their movements may appear _____ and _____ .

11. _____ behavior such as the repeated checking and adjusting can signal stress.

12. If your fellow diver is unable to recognize you or react to your presence, beware; severe _____ may be present and _____ could result.

13. If your own breathing becomes rapid and shallow, _____ and _____ about what is bothering you and what you need to do to regain _____ .

14. In over _____ of diving fatalities, the victim failed to _____ the _____ .

15. Gaining buoyancy at the surface should be an _____ _____ ; a contingency skill for additional buoyancy at the surface is _____ _____ .

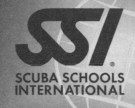

PART 2
Rescue

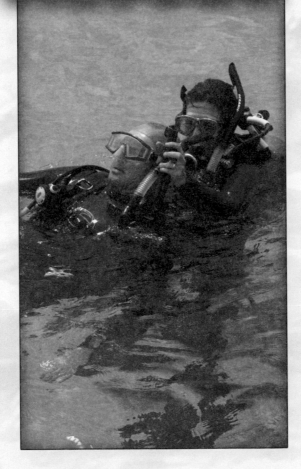

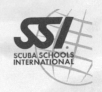

Accident
Management

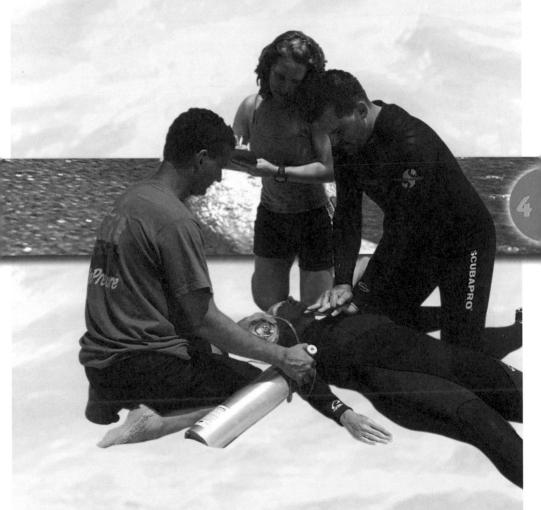

Managing Accidents

In Sections 2 and 3 we discussed what causes stress and how it can be prevented, as well as how to detect and deal with stress throughout the diving process. When stress is identified and contained, panic and accident situations can be avoided. However, what happens when you are not able to stop stress in your buddy from escalating, either because of its sudden occurrence, or because of buddy separation? In this instance you may need to step in as a rescue diver and take charge of the situation. It may include searching for your buddy, or it may include recovering their unconscious body from the water. You should be prepared for these situations, both physically and mentally.

Section 4 Objectives
After completing this section you will be able to:

◆ Understand the Accident Management process,

◆ Describe common signs and symptoms of diving maladies,

◆ List the first aid procedures for diving emergencies.

While physical skill will help you carry out a buddy rescue, mental stamina is what will carry both you and the victim through the accident until professional medical assistance arrives.

This process can be defined as accident management, or your ability to control yourself, the victim, the surrounding witnesses, and the emergency personnel during a buddy rescue.

Below is a list of the basic accident management techniques that a rescue diver should know:

♦ Emergency procedures and contacts

♦ Coordinating rescue personnel

♦ Knowing the limits of your abilities and when to get help

♦ Keeping a written record of the accident and treatment

♦ Searching for a missing diver

♦ Rescuing an accident victim

♦ Checking the victim's vital signs including pulse and respiration

♦ Recognizing the symptoms of compressed gas injuries

♦ Providing first aid, CPR, and oxygen administration to the victim

♦ Providing psychological support to the victim and the witnesses

♦ Transporting or evacuating the victim

While prevention of stress will always be your number one priority when diving, preparation in the area of accident management may be the life-saving difference in a panic or rescue situation.

Emergency Procedures and Contacts

Before you leave for your dive destination, you should prepare a list of emergency procedures and numbers using the SSI Accident Management Slate. You should know who to contact in the region where you'll be diving in case of an emergency, and know the location of the nearest emergency medical facility. Check the qualifications and communication capabilities of the resort or charter operation. Do they have a predetermined plan for dealing with injured divers? Is there an airlift operation available?

If a planned destination does not have adequate safety support, you may want to change your plans. The simple confidence a safe dive location provides can contribute to a stress-free dive. Once you reach your diving location or board your boat, you may want to check out the communication and emergency equipment so you know where they are located and how they operate. Through this extra preparation you will be able to help in case of an emergency.

▲ VICTIM'S NAME

▲ ADDRESS

▲ PHONE NUMBER

▲ DATE / TIME

▲ ALLERGIES

▲ MEDICATIONS

▲ IN CASE OF EMERGENCY, CONTACT

▲ LOCAL MEDICAL FACILITY

Emergency Contact Information.

Included in your written list should be the phone number of the nearest emergency medical service (EMS). Be sure to have enough coins to make phone calls. It is also a good idea to let your buddy know about any past medical history which may be of interest to medical personnel, such as previous decompression sickness, blood sugar disorders, recent surgery, and drug allergies. All this information should be kept accessible; you might want to affix it to the inside cover of your log book, for instance, and let your buddy know about it.

Accessibility to First Responder Equipment

First responder equipment should be available in the area where you are diving. If diving locally, you may simply need to know who to contact for help such as the fire

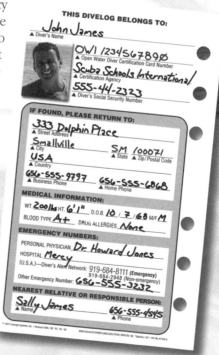

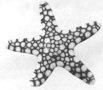

department, lifeguard station, Coast Guard, hospital, police, or the local Dive Rescue Team. Regardless of the availability of medical and rescue personnel, there are a few items that need to be immediately accessible. First, we'll list those which you are definitely accountable for, and then we'll list those which you may want to provide if not already available:

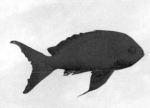

What You Need	*What Should be Immediately Available*
✓ Access to telephone/radio	✓ 100% oxygen
✓ Whistle	✓ Radio (CB or VHF)
✓ First aid kit	✓ Binoculars
✓ First aid booklet	✓ Lines (100 feet/30 metres) and stuff sack
✓ Blankets	
✓ Underwater compass	✓ Marker buoys
✓ Clipboard, paper and pen	✓ Surf or rescue board

If your local diving area isn't set up for emergencies, you should contact a national group such as DAN (Divers Alert Network) in the United States or the DES (Divers Emergency Service) in the South Pacific for advice on how to proceed and who to contact in your area.

Coordinating Rescue Personnel

In the event of an accident, you, as a rescue diver, will need to coordinate any available personnel on the scene to help with the rescue. If there is someone more qualified on the scene, make yourself available and follow directions. If no one else takes charge or is available to help, it is up to you to lead the rescue.

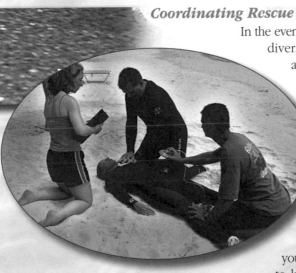

A rescue diver must take control of the accident scene.

At the beginning of your dive trip, you should get to know the other people in your group to find out what their various backgrounds are. Mentally note if they would be able to help during an emergency. Many doctors, paramedics, and other emergency personnel are frequently divers. By getting to know your fellow divers, you should also get a feeling for who could be used in a rescue situation.

Should you ever find yourself in charge of a diver rescue, be it your own buddy or a fellow diver, you must remain calm and in mental control. Your strength will keep the group under control and prevent chaos on the scene. You will need to make quick and decisive decisions. Assign duties based on the number of available personnel. Ideally you will need two divers in the water to help rescue the victim, one person on shore to control the search pattern, one bystander to go and get help, and possibly one observer to keep track of the victim in the water. Ideally, you should also have a recorder who can write down what is occurring on the accident scene.

Weighing the Situation

If you are ever in a rescue situation by yourself, you will need to weigh the benefits vs. the risks between attempting the rescue and immediate care, whether you should get help, and at what point.

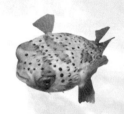

Backup support is a good reason to dive in a group, especially if inexperienced divers are present, or if you are making a potentially risky dive. Knowing you have people to rely on can lower stress in itself, and having people to help out can make the difference between a successful and unsuccessful rescue.

Knowing the Limits of Your Abilities

Because mental strength is as important to a rescue as preparation, you will need to constantly monitor yourself and know when you have reached the limits of your abilities. You will be responsible for providing psychological support to the victim, the rescuers, and the witnesses. Any breakdown on your part may affect the smooth operation of the rescue.

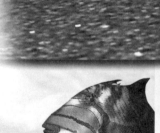

When you begin to tire, lack the ability to make decisions, or lend support, it is time to get help. Whether it is simply turning your responsibility over to another diver or calling for assistance, know when the time is right.

You may also lack the experience to lead a successful search pattern off a dive boat. Instead of pushing your chances, wait and call for assistance rather than jeopardizing your's or another's safety. Never compromise your, or anyone else's, safety during a rescue attempt.

Keeping a Written Record

If possible, assign someone to record the rescue proceedings so you have an accurate record of how the accident occurred and the treatment that followed. This will help the emergency rescue personnel administer further treatment, and will also aid in any follow-up investigation (should one occur).

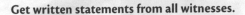

Get written statements from all witnesses.

Get a written statement from the victim's dive buddy (if you are not the buddy), as well as all the witnesses as to what caused the accident. Write down what rescue procedures were followed, who was in charge of each phase of the rescue, and what immediate care was given. You may wish to either turn the report over to the emergency services personnel, or you may want to accompany the victim to the hospital so you can report first hand. Your thorough reporting will help the victim receive better care, and will cover your involvement in the accident should an investigation occur.

Searching for a Missing Diver

Should you or another diver surface without a buddy, you will need to begin a search pattern in an attempt to locate him/her as quickly as possible. As the rescue leader, you will have to weigh the risk/benefit factor of a search pattern, or in other words, does the benefit of the search outweigh the possible risks. Your decision should be based on the weather conditions, how long the diver has been missing, if you have a specific location to search, and how much diver support is available to aid in the search.

When there is a chance to save a life — a rescue mode operation — then the potential benefit will be considered high. The dive team responding in rescue mode, with a potentially high benefit, will be able to justify a certain amount of risk.[1]

[1]Steven J. Linton, Damon A. Rust & T. Daniel Gilliam, *Dive Rescue Specialist Training Manual* (Fort Collins: Concept Systems, 1986), p. 24

If you feel that a search pattern should be instigated, proceed quickly yet safely. Actual equipment and procedures for search patterns are covered in more detail in Section 5, Rescue Skills.

Rescuing an Accident Victim

When rescuing an accident victim, whether conscious or unconscious, you will need to get them to the surface and out of the water as quickly as possible. It is impossible to administer immediate care while the victim is still in the water. The skills that are needed to rescue an accident victim are covered in detail in Section 5, Rescue Skills.

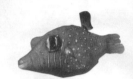

Checking Vital Signs

In any life-threatening emergency, the person administering first aid must be able to evaluate the victim's condition and respond accordingly. Most importantly is whether or not the person is breathing and has a pulse. The easiest way to check a victim's vital signs is to use the first aid ABC's.

A = Airway:
Be sure there are no obstructions.

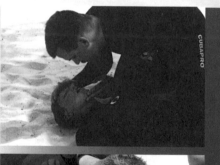

B = Breathing:
If the victim is not breathing, open airway and give 2 quick breaths.

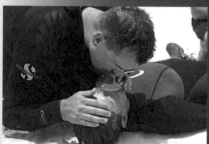

C = Circulation:
Check pulse. If there is no heartbeat, begin CPR.

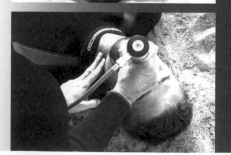

To check if the victim is breathing, listen and look for the chest to rise and fall; if not, begin rescue breathing. Rescue breathing can be given in the water if a pulse is present, and you feel it will increase the victim's chance of survival. If your victim has no pulse, once you have him/her on a hard surface begin CPR and do not stop until either the pulse is restored, someone else alternates with you, you become exhausted, or medical personnel arrive to take over. Never attempt CPR in the water.

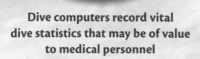

If the water is cold, you are wearing gloves, or the victim is wearing a hood and/or dry suit, it may be very difficult to check the victim's vital signs in the water. If so, you should get the victim back to the boat or shore immediately so you can remove the obstructive clothing and check the victim's ABC's.

If the victim is conscious, it's important to get an idea of what he perceives to be the problem. Listening to what he says can give you a fairly accurate idea of what is going on, and he'll probably volunteer more information than you thought to ask for.

Find out as much information about the dive itself as you can. What was the profile, and how reliable is the information that the victim gave you? Were there any problems associated with the dive? How was the victim feeling before the dive? Preserve his/her equipment just as it was when he/she took it off. If the victim was using a dive computer, send it along to the treatment facility, they may be able to retrieve information from it. If the diver is unconscious or suffering from symptoms, have another diver gather this information while you begin treatment and transportation of the diver. Regardless of the type of symptoms the diver is experiencing, he/she should go to the nearest medical facility for further evaluation.[2]

Dive computers record vital dive statistics that may be of value to medical personnel

[2]Kathy R.N. Work, *Med Dive Textbook* (Fort Collins: Dive Rescue Inc./International, 1990), p. 48

Recognizing Compressed Gas Injuries

As you learned in your Open Water Diver Course, breathing compressed gasses under water opens the diver up to a variety of diving maladies based on the effects of increasing and decreasing pressure. As a diving buddy and rescue diver, you should be able to understand the causes of compressed gas injuries, as well as recognize the symptoms. If you are able to detect the symptoms, you can relay this information to emergency personnel who may not be educated in diving maladies.

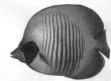

Your early identification and immediate treatment can save a life, and help avoid permanent neurological damage to the victim.

Immediate care for diving injuries is covered in detail later in this section.

If a compressed gas injury is suspected, administer the 5-minute neuro-exam as covered in the appendix of this book (pg. A-4), or as shown on your SSI Diving Accident Management Slate.

Decompression Sickness

To avoid decompression sickness (DCS) always adhere to dive computer or the SSI dive tables and never push their limits. Do not make decompression dives unless you are trained to do them, and be conservative with multi-day, multi-level, repetitive diving. Over half of the DCS victims reported to the Divers Alert Network were performing either repetitive or multi-day dives. Also, be aware that age, fatigue, body weight, alcohol consumption, dehydration and other unknown factors can cause some divers to be more susceptible to decompression sickness, even when no-decompression limits are strictly adhered to.

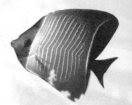

Signs and Symptoms of Decompression Sickness:

◆ Tingling and itching of the skin

◆ Blotchy skin rash

◆ Local pain in arms, legs and joints

◆ Dizziness

◆ Loss of Coordination

◆ Unusual fatigue or weakness

◆ Numbness and paralysis

◆ Shortness of breath and coughing spasms

◆ Collapse or unconsciousness

Decompression sickness symptoms usually appear between 15 minutes and 12 hours after surfacing from a dive; but in severe cases they may appear sooner. Delayed occurrence (over 24 hours) is rare, but can occur, especially if air travel follows diving. Delaying or failing to seek treatment is probably one of the worst things the injured diver can do. Some treatment delays may be due to unavoidable situations, such as remote or inaccessible dive sites. But all too often the delay is caused by fears, misconceptions, or just plain denial on the part of the diver. In fact, the Divers Alert Network reports that only 37% of divers who experienced DCS got treatment within 12 hours after the symptoms appeared.[3]

As a rescue diver, you must be able to help recognize the symptoms of DCS and get the diver immediate care as quickly as possible. As with all compressed gas injuries, the quicker and more aggressive the treatment, the lower the chances of permanent damage to the diver.

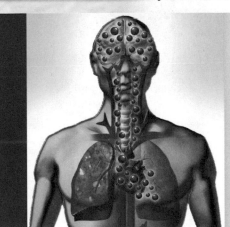

Air Embolism

If a diver fails to exhale when ascending, the air trapped in the lungs will expand, rupturing the lungs and allowing air to escape into the bloodstream and body tissue. Air bubbles in the bloodstream can restrict blood flow to the brain and eventually lead to unconsciousness and paralysis. Signs and symptoms of an air embolism usually appear during or immediately after surfacing and may resemble those of a stroke.

[3]Kathy R.N. Work, *Med Dive Textbook* (Fort Collins: Dive Rescue Inc./International, 1990), p. 50

According to the Divers Alert Network, air embolism sometimes occurs unexpectedly in divers who ascend normally but have lung conditions which result in local air trapping. Although most lung diseases can cause this problem, some common conditions are the following: lung infections, lung cysts, tumors, scar tissue, mucous plugs, and obtrusive lung diseases. The diver may not be aware of the risk because some of these conditions are undetectable even with a medical examination. There are no breathing maneuvers which will decrease the risk of embolism if the diver has one of these disorders.[4]

Signs and Symptoms of Air Embolism:

- Dizziness
- Visual blurring
- Chest pain
- Personality change
- Paralysis or weakness
- Bloody froth from the mouth or nose
- Convulsions and distortion
- Unconsciousness
- Respiratory failure

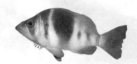

Pneumothorax

Pneumothorax is another lung overexpansion problem. It occurs when air escapes into the space between the lung and the chest cavity and then expands, causing a lung collapse. Pneumothorax does not require recompression, but does require medical treatment to release air from the chest cavity and reinflate the lung.

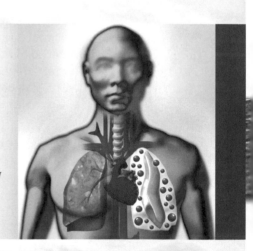

Signs and Symptoms of Pneumothorax:

- Respiratory distress
- Sharp pain in chest
- Blue skin, lips, and fingernails
- Rapid heartbeat

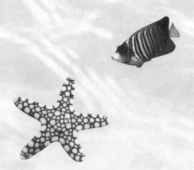

[4]G. Yancey Mebane M.D. & Arthur P. Dick M.D., *Underwater Diving Accident Manual* (Durham: Duke UP, 1985), p. 17

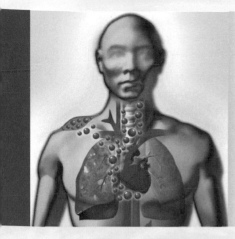

Mediastinal Emphysema and Subcutaneous Emphysema

Mediastinal emphysema results when air becomes trapped in the cavity between the lungs and around the heart.

Subcutaneous emphysema has the same cause as air embolism but the results are not as serious. Air escapes into the tissues underneath the skin, usually near the neck or collar bone.

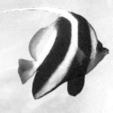

Signs and Symptoms of Mediastinal Emphysema

◆ Pain in chest, usually under breastbone

◆ Difficulty in breathing

◆ Faintness

◆ Change in voice

Signs and Symptoms of Subcutaneous Emphysema

◆ Difficulty in breathing and swallowing

◆ Change in sound of voice

◆ Swelling around face, neck, and upper chest

◆ Crackling sensation when skin is touched

Administering Immediate Care

In a suspected diving accident the first question is, "Did the victim take a breath under water?" Based on that question, an Immediate Care Protocol has been developed by the Divers Alert Network to assist in determining the proper actions to take. This Protocol is shown in detail on the next page.

If the injured diver did not breathe under water, the problem is not a pressure-related injury. Give appropriate first aid as necessary, such as CPR and 100% oxygen, and activate the local emergency medical system.

If the injured diver did breathe under water, determine if the symptoms are mild or serious. For mild symptoms, administer appropriate first aid and 100% oxygen, and activate the emergency medical system. For serious symptoms, the victim requires emergency medical treatment as quickly as possible. Follow the same basic first aid procedures as mild symptoms but activate the emergency medical system as quickly as possible.

When evaluating a victim's symptoms there are two serious compressed gas injuries that are life threatening: decompression sickness and air embolism. In the field, for first aid purposes, they may be grouped together as decompression illness (DCI), as they both require the same basic steps. So, if a victim shows signs of either decompression sickness or air embolism, it is not necessary to distinguish which is occurring; treat it as decompression illness.

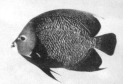

The following Immediate Care Protocol is reprinted with permission from the DAN Dive & Travel Guide (G.Y. Mebane, M.D., editor)

1. **Provide cardiopulmonary resuscitation (CPR) if needed.**

2. **Did diver have a source of compressed air or other breathing gas under water?**

   a. No
      - ◆ Probably not a decompression illness
      - ◆ Give appropriate first aid
      - ◆ Call for help if needed

   b. Yes
      - ◆ Decompression illness must be considered a cause
      - ◆ Follow this protocol and give appropriate first aid
      - ◆ Call for help in management and evacuation

3. **Did symptoms begin while diver was under water?**
   - ◆ Always serious
   - ◆ Begin treatment for serious symptoms

4. **Are the symptoms mild? (see above)**
   - ◆ Severe fatigue
   - ◆ Itching not related to marine or aquatic life
   - ◆ Non-painful joint "awareness"

5. If only mild symptoms are present:

◆ Place diver in lateral recumbent (recovery) position (see page 4-17)

◆ Make brief neurological assessment (do not allow to interfere with urgent first aid measures)

◆ Begin oxygen first aid (use 100% oxygen delivered by a demand inhalator system or non-rebreather mask — see page 4-16)

◆ Protect diver from heat, cold, further injury

◆ Evaluate for other illness or injury in addition to DCI

6. If mild symptoms are present:

◆ Observe carefully for improvement or worsening

◆ Continue oxygen as long as available

If symptoms are still present treat as serious:

◆ If symptoms resolve, continue oxygen and observe

◆ Contact DAN or EMS for assistance

7. If serious symptoms are present (see bottom of this page):

◆ Maintain appropriate position

◆ Continue oxygen as long as available

◆ Constant observation and periodic neurological evaluation

◆ Maintain contact with Coast Guard, Rescue Squad or other emergency agency

◆ Contact DAN when possible

8. If serious symptoms improve or clear completely:

◆ Continue oxygen and other measures

◆ Evacuate to medical facility as soon as possible

9. If serious symptoms are not improving or are getting worse:

◆ Carefully recheck techniques of first aid and make corrections needed

◆ Notify emergency agency of situation

◆ Make an urgent evacuation consistent with safety

Mild vs. Serious Symptoms

Whether a diver has mild or serious symptoms determines the first aid administered and the action taken, as is shown in the Immediate Care Protocol. According to DAN, mild symptoms are warning signs, and include fatigue and itching. Joint pain is sometimes considered a mild sign, but should be treated as a scrious symptom. Serious symptoms are medical emergencies, and include pain, weakness, dizziness, numbness, or decreased consciousness. Recognizing the symptoms of diving injuries, and whether they are mild or serious, can help save divers.

Administering Oxygen

Oxygen works in several ways to help the injured diver, and is probably the most important aspect of treatment, other than recompression. It can produce dramatic reversals in the diver's condition, even relieving severe symptoms such as paralysis. But it must be stressed that oxygen does not replace the need for recompression, and discontinuing its use can cause symptoms to return.[5]

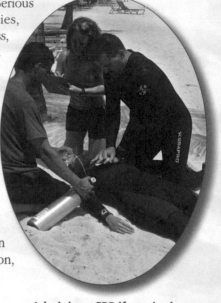

Administer CPR if required.

According to DAN, administering oxygen to a conscious, spontaneously breathing diver is not difficult and is considered the standard of care. However, if the victim is unconscious or not breathing spontaneously, oxygen administration becomes more complicated. In this situation the rescuer must have an understanding of airway management and the use of oxygen equipment. In addition, rescuers should also be aware that there may be various state laws or regulations dealing with the use of 100% oxygen.[6]

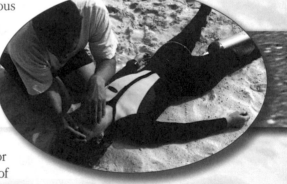

The person administering oxygen should be trained in the use of oxygen equipment.

Although the benefits of 100% oxygen have been proven, and it is difficult to further injure a diver with oxygen, it is recommended that the person administering the oxygen be trained in the use of oxygen equipment and airway management. If your boat or dive group does not provide oxygen on site, you should know where to easily access it. Check with your local SSI Authorized Dive Center about courses in your local area.

[5]Kathy R.N. Work, *Med Dive Textbook* (Fort Collins: Dive Rescue Inc./International, 1990, p. 59
[6]G. Yancey Mebane M.D., editor. *DAN Dive & Travel Medical Guide.* (Durham: Divers Alert Network, 1995), p. 12

Positioning the Injured Diver

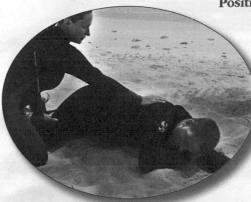

When positioning injured divers, consider the severity of their symptoms. Fully alert divers with minor symptoms, who are not in distress, can be positioned horizontally. Keep them comfortable and make sure that the blood flow is not obstructed. Examples of possible blood-flow obstructions include crossed legs and the head resting on arms. According to the Divers Alert Network, "inert gas elimination is still occurring and obstructed blood flow to an extremity will interfere with off-gassing."

If a diver experiences mild symptoms, DAN recommends the lateral recumbent (recovery) position.

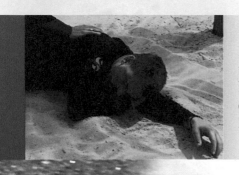

If a diver experiences mild symptoms after surfacing, the Divers Alert Network recommends the lateral recumbent (recovery) position. In this position, the diver is on the side, head supported, with the upper leg bent at the knee.

Divers with serious symptoms, such as intense headache, severe pain, weakness or paralysis, may change in the level of consciousness and require a more controlled position. There is danger that they may become worse as time passes, and a very frequent occurrence is nausea and vomiting. Divers should be in a position so that the airway will not be blocked if vomiting occurs.

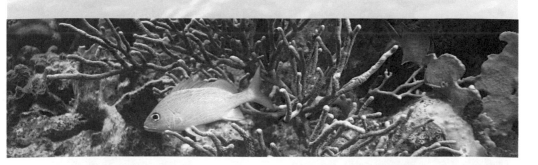

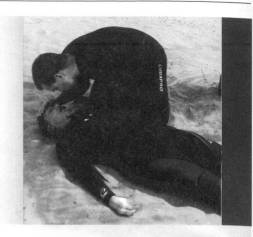

Of course, if ventilatory or cardiac resuscitation is required, the injured diver must be supine (on the back, face upward). Vomiting in this position is extremely dangerous; if it occurs, the diver should be quickly turned to the side until the airway is cleared and resuscitation can resume in the supine position.

Providing Psychological Support

An accident can produce heated emotions that will need to be contained in order to keep the scene under control. Both the victim and the witnesses may undergo stress, especially if the witness is a related party such as a husband or wife. The situation will require patience, compassion and tact. If the witnesses are in control, use them to help out. Keeping busy will many times keep your mind off the severity of the situation. If the witnesses are emotional or irrational you may want them out of the scene, yet informed of the progress.

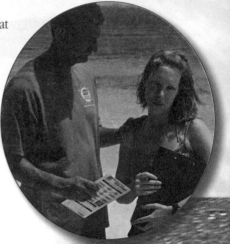

A rescue diver may need to lend psychological support at the accident scene.

If there are enough people on location, you may want someone to sit with emotional witnesses to keep them under control.

You will also need to lend emotional support to the accident victim. Let them know that everything is OK and that help is on the way. Keep the victim involved in the treatment, asking questions, and keeping their mind alert. Don't allow them to dwell on the negativity of the situation. Keep them informed and don't talk to others as if they cannot hear. A smile and a reassuring pat on the back will keep up a positive attitude.

Transporting and Evacuating the Victim

When it comes time to transport the victim to an emergency medical facility, you will need to determine the best method of transportation. Your decision should be based on the distance to the facility and the severity of the injury. Ground transportation is the most common and the safest method. When a diver with a compressed gas injury is taken to altitude, such as when flying, they are subjected to decreasing ambient pressure and the possibility that the nitrogen may come out of solution, or, in the case of an embolism, that the existing air bubbles in the system may expand, causing further damage.

If the medical facility is far and time is of the essence, you may have little choice but to airlift the victim.

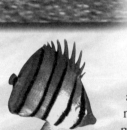

If the medical facility is far, and time is of the essence, you may have little choice but to airlift the victim, most probably by helicopter.

During an air evacuation, the pilot is in charge of all aspects of the aircraft operation, while medical personnel on board supervise the actual care of the patient. As a rescue diver, your most important job as a ground crew will be to secure the landing zone. If you are on a boat with no deck, you may need to tow a dinghy or raft behind you. This will give the helicopter a more accessible area to pick up the victim. If the evacuation is at night, you will need to light up the landing zone as much as possible, spot lighting any obstructions the helicopter will need to see. On the boat, secure the zone by lowering any masts, booms or antennas. On a boat or solid ground, any loose debris such as paper and equipment should be cleared away. In any evacuation situation, follow all orders from the aircraft crew on how to hoist the victim. Each situation may warrant different safety and evacuation procedures.

In addition to knowing how to contact help, all rescue divers should be properly trained in first aid and CPR. If you are with an accident victim you may need to administer first aid, rescue breathing, or CPR until help arrives. The importance of basic first aid and CPR skills for all individuals involved in aquatic activities cannot be overly stressed.

Summary

When turning a victim over to emergency personnel you should be able to relate to them the details of the accident, the probable injury, and the immediate care as registered in your written accident record. In other words, as a rescue diver you should be able to recognize the symptoms of decompression sickness and air embolism, for instance, so that you can expedite emergency care. Proper accident management skills and preparation will carry both you and the victim through the accident until professional medical assistance arrives.

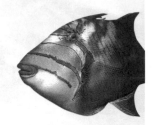

In Section 5 we will look more in detail at the rescue skills you will need to perform a buddy assist or buddy rescue, as well as how to rescue an unconscious diver.

Section 4 Review Questions

1. Before you leave for your dive destination, you should prepare a list of _____ _____ and _____ using the SSI Accident Management Slate.

2. In the event of an accident, you, as a rescue diver, will need to _____ any available _____ on the scene to help with the rescue.

3. Your strength will keep the group under _____ and prevent _____ on the scene.

4. You will be responsible for providing _____ support to the _____ , the _____ , and the _____ .

5. If possible, assign someone to record the rescue _____ so you have an accurate _____ of how the accident occurred and the _____ that followed.

6. As the rescue leader, you will have to weigh the risk/benefit factor of a _____ _____ , or in other words, does the benefit of the search outweigh the possible risks.

7. The easiest way to check a victim's vital signs is to use the first aid _____ .

8. If the victim was using a _____ _____ , send it along to the treatment facility, they may be able to retrieve information from it.

9. As a rescue diver, you must be able to help recognize the symptoms of DCS and get the diver _____ _____ as quickly as possible.

10. According to the Divers Alert Network, air embolism sometimes occurs unexpectedly in divers who _____ normally but have _____ conditions which result in local air trapping.

11. In a suspected diving accident the first question is, " _____ _____ ?"

12. _____ works in several ways to help the injured diver, and is probably the most important aspect of _____ , other than _____ .

13. Although the benefits of _____ % oxygen have been proven, and it is difficult to further injure a diver with oxygen, it is recommended that the person administering the oxygen be _____ in the use of oxygen equipment and airway management.

14. If a diver experiences mild symptoms after surfacing, the Divers Alert Network recommends the _____ _____ _____ position.

15. You will also need to lend _____ support to the _____ _____ .

SCUBA SCHOOLS
INTERNATIONAL

Rescue
Skills

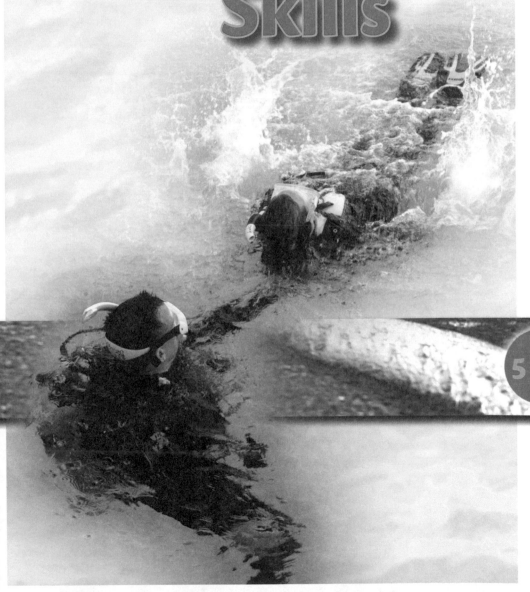

5

Though our emphasis in this text is on early detection of stress to prevent accidents, 100 percent avoidance is impossible. Diving accidents have many extenuating circumstances and are usually caused by a combination of problems. But even when panic or an accident has occurred, the accompanying stress can be dealt with so that rescue can be dealt with through self-aid, buddy assist, buddy rescue, or at last resort, by rescuing an unconscious diver.

As in any advanced diving course each participant has a different background and has been trained to perform skills in slightly different ways. We do not intend to overrule your training methods, but rather to adapt your existing skills to a competence in rescue training.

Section 5 Objectives

After completing this section you will be able to describe the skills needed to:

◆ Provide "self-aid,"

◆ Provide assistance to your buddy,

◆ Perform a buddy rescue,

◆ Perform an unconscious-diver rescue.

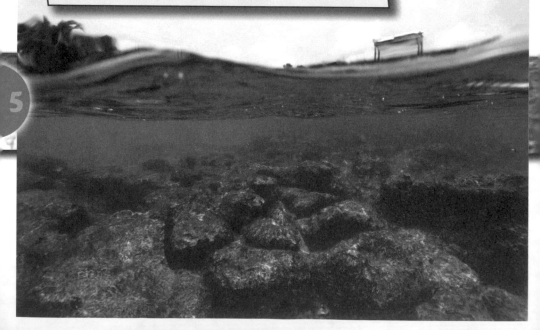

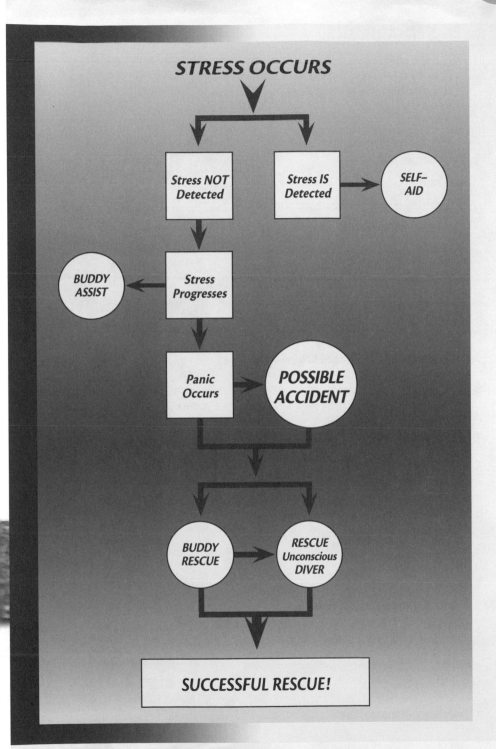

Progression of Stress to a Rescue Situation.

Self-Aid

The skills needed for self-aid are basically the same skills learned in an Open Water Diver course. Many are used in every diving situation; others would only be used in an emergency.

Skills Needed for Self-Aid

1. **Buoyancy control**
   a. Remaining neutrally buoyant under water
   b. Controlling buoyancy on ascents and descents
   c. Using positive buoyancy to rest at the surface

2. **Survival swimming techniques**
   a. Swimming
   b. Bobbing or floating
   c. Treading water or swimming in place

3. **Using alternate fin kicks when tired**
   a. Scissor kick
   b. Dolphin kick

4. **Relieving leg cramps**

5. **Switching breathing methods as needed**
   a. Mouth
   b. Snorkel
   c. Regulator
   d. Alternate air source

6. **Mask and second-stage regulator clearing, and second-stage regulator retrieval**

7. **Taking off, adjusting, and replacing gear**
   a. On the surface
   b. Under water

8. **Emergency swimming ascent**

9. **Emergency buoyant ascent and weight ditching**

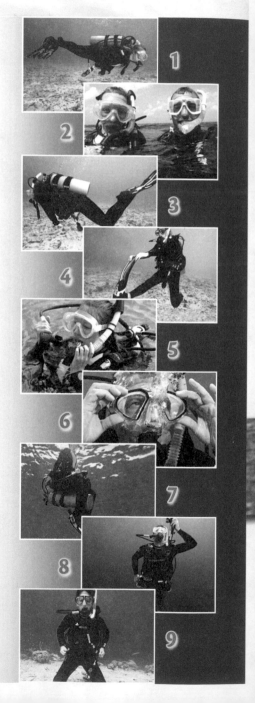

Stop-Breathe-Think-Act

In any emergency situation you need to regain control before you act. The best way to regain control quickly is to immediately stop, calm down, and take several deep breaths. This will relax you and help you make a rational decision, and also prevent an irrational decision that might be dangerous. Once under control, you can weigh the alternatives and choose the appropriate action.

Of course, this whole process should only take a few seconds because in an emergency, time is of the essence. An out-of-air situation is the most critical and demands immediate attention, but in most cases, "stop-breathe-think-act" is the best way to regain control and make an intelligent decision.

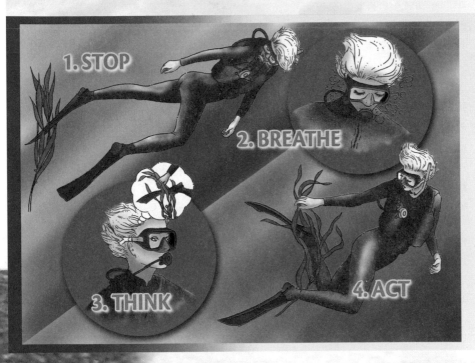

1. STOP
2. BREATHE
3. THINK
4. ACT

Buddy Assist

A buddy assist is used when a buddy is experiencing stress but is still under control. In such a case, a helping hand from a buddy may be all that is needed to remedy the problem. As a buddy, you can help your partner perform a self-aid skill such as relieving a leg cramp. Be alert so that you can detect the problem, and communicate so that you can determine how to assist. If you are familiar with your buddy's equipment, such as how the power inflator operates, a buddy assist will run smoother. Most skills are performed better with help, so in addition to offering assistance, ask for help whenever it is necessary.

As many of the skills needed for a buddy assist are similar to those for self-aid, only those that go beyond your original open water training are covered in detail.

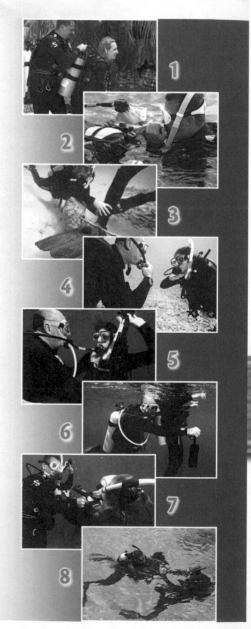

Skills Needed for Buddy Assists

1. **Helping your buddy hold, remove, and replace gear**
   a. Under water
   b. On the surface

2. **Inflating your buddy's BC**
   a. Oral inflation
   b. Power inflation

3. **Helping a buddy who is entangled or entrapped**

4. **Responding to your buddy's hand signals**

5. **Alternate air source breathing and ascents**

6. **Ditching your buddy's equipment**

7. **Buoyancy control**
   a. Maintaining neutral buoyancy
   b. Controlling ascents and descents
   c. Positive buoyancy on the surface

8. **Towing your buddy**

Entanglement in kelp, nets, fishing line, or coral can be a major source of stress for the diver. This constriction of movement can be serious enough to require a buddy's assistance. Remember to remain calm during an entanglement situation. Struggling will only lead to further entanglement.

To help your buddy, calmly untangle him or her if possible, and resort to cutting with your diver's tool only if necessary, being careful not to damage the environment if it is at all avoidable. Another way to get out of an entanglement is to remove the scuba unit while keeping the second-stage regulator in your mouth. This can be accomplished on your own, but as with any self-aid skill, it is easier when assisted by a buddy.

Entrapment

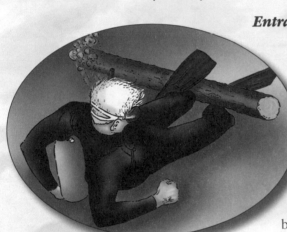

Although entrapment is rare, you should know how to help a diver in this situation. The biggest concern is air supply, and getting fresh air to the diver until you can get him or her free. Keep the diver calm through constant communication, and should you need to return to the surface for help, be sure your buddy knows where you are going and that you will be back.

The biggest concern with an entrapped diver is air supply.

If any other divers are present, use their help. If you need to return to the surface, make sure a diver stays with your buddy. If you must leave air with your entrapped buddy, forfeit your air supply and make an air sharing ascent with one of the other divers. Be sure and note the exact location of the entrapment so you will be able to relocate your buddy quickly.

Towing Your Buddy

If your buddy becomes fatigued and is unable to swim back to the boat or shore without risking exhaustion, you may want to help with a simple tow. First we'll list some important points in making a tow safe and effective, then we'll go on to discuss four common methods of towing.

♦ Choose the tow that is safest and easiest for the environment and situation.

♦ Make yourself and your buddy positively buoyant.

♦ Keep your buddy's face above water, and use your own snorkel or second-stage regulator as conditions require.

♦ Keep your buddy at or near the horizontal position in the water so that you have freedom to swim and kick.

♦ Stay in constant communication with your buddy, providing encouragement and reassurance.

♦ Ditch any extra equipment that hinders the tow, such as goody bags, game, cameras, cylinders, etc.

♦ Have your buddy help by doing an easy kick if possible.

♦ Change positions, fin kicks, or method of towing to relieve or avoid muscle fatigue.

Towing Beside Your Buddy

Side-by-side towing is the most common method and should be used with calm divers. To perform this tow, hold your buddy by placing your arm through his or her underarm. The physical and visual contact provided by this tow gives your buddy a sense of security. Hold on to your buddy with your closest hand, then swim side-by-side, with the buddy lying back. Your body will be horizontal but slightly sideways in the water, requiring a scissors kick. From this position you will be able to monitor your buddy and stay in constant communication.

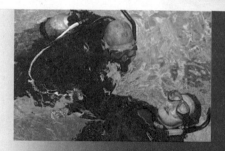
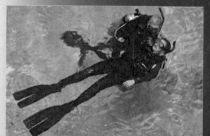
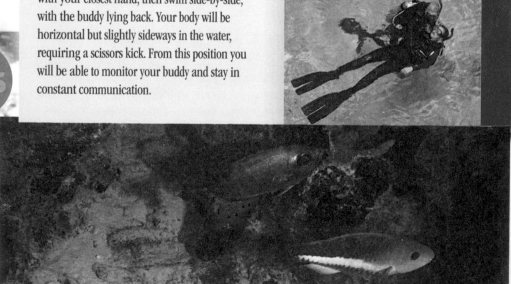

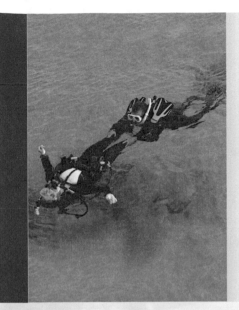

Towing Your Buddy From the Feet

This tow works well with calm divers because it allows the victim to float on his or her back and relax in the water. To perform the tow, have your buddy lie back in the water and place his or her fins against your shoulders. Then hold on to your buddy's knees and push him or her along as you swim. This tow allows you to swim comfortably on your stomach, allows you to see where you are going, and lets you communicate with your buddy. It is also a good tow to use when there is a long distance to cover; buddies can take turns being towed to conserve energy.

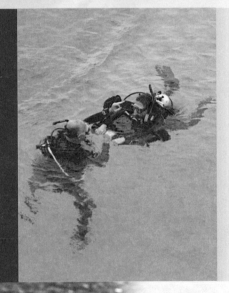

Towing Your Buddy with a Surface Float

A surface float, or any other piece of equipment, can be used for either a calm or panicking diver. A calm diver simply holds on to the float as you tow it. This method allows the victim to either stay down in the water, breathing through the snorkel or second-stage regulator, or to elevate the chest to keep the head above water. The surface float works with a panicked diver because it keeps you and the victim separated, and allows the victim to rest with their head above water so they can relax and get under control.

5

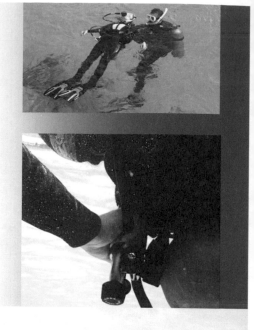

Towing Your Buddy From Behind

This is the least popular method and is used mainly when a victim is panicking and a surface float or other equipment is not available. To perform the tow from behind, have the victim lie back in the water while you hold onto his or her cylinder, BC, or wet suit. This keeps you out of reach, but it also requires that you swim backwards. From this position it is difficult to maintain direction, and allows no eye contact to reassure a victim.

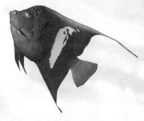

Procedures to Protect Yourself and Perform a Buddy Assist

In a buddy assist, your buddy should be able to remain in physical and mental control, but the situation can escalate at any time, so be prepared. Always remember to take care of yourself first–without your safety, both of your lives could become endangered. Few assists do, however, turn into panic situations. Usually, if you are there to help, panic can be avoided. The following eight steps are suggested procedure to follow in a buddy assist situation:

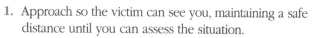

1. Approach so the victim can see you, maintaining a safe distance until you can assess the situation.

2. Make physical contact and speak to your buddy.

3. Attempt to find out what is causing the problem.

4. Stop, breathe, think and communicate — get yourself under control.

5. Proceed slowly, using the available equipment to assist you.

6. Once on the surface establish positive buoyancy. Ditch your buddy's weight if necessary.

7. Use the best breathing method for surface conditions.

8. Help your buddy to the exit point with a simple tow if necessary.

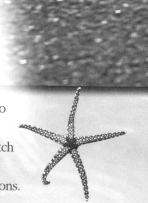

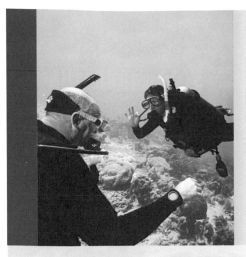

Approach so the Victim Can See You

It will help your buddy to calm down when he or she sees you and to gain confidence because of your attempt to help. If you are unsure about your buddy's mental state, stop out of reach until you can assess the situation. Eye contact and communication through hand signals can calm most buddies in distress. If you must leave or move out of sight, let your buddy know what you are doing and when you will return.

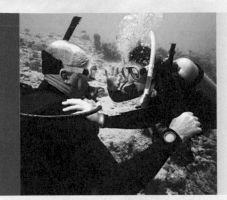

Make Physical Contact

Once you have decided it is necessary to approach your buddy, you should make physical contact. If you are on the surface, establish positive buoyancy first in case your buddy becomes aggressive. In most cases a firm grip or a pat on the back will calm a distressed diver.

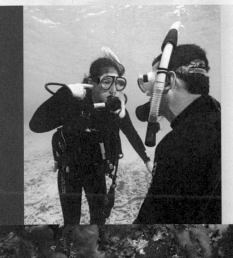

Find Out What is Causing the Problem

In order to solve a problem, you need to understand the cause. Examine your buddy to determine the source of stress. Is he entangled? Is a piece of equipment lost or malfunctioning? Is his ear not clearing properly? Or is he simply fatigued? Through observation and a few simple questions you should be able to sort out the problem and determine the proper solution.

5

Stop-Breathe-Think-Communicate

You must get yourself under control before you can help others. If you feel your stress level increase because of your buddy's predicament, stop, breathe deeply and calm down. Then instruct your buddy to do the same. Deep breathing will help calm both of you down. Once you have calmed down think about the proper solution and communicate it to your buddy. In a buddy assist you have the luxury of time because it is not yet an emergency.

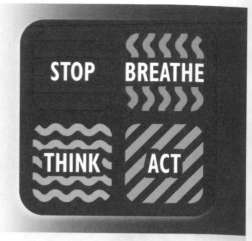

Proceed Slowly, Using Available Equipment to Assist You

Once you have decided on the solution, you are ready to act. Drop any equipment that interferes, and utilize any equipment that can aid the assist. The compass, BC, knife, and alternate air source are some of the pieces that might assist you. If you feel that surfacing is the best solution, let your inflation system help you. Learn to let equipment do as much of the work as possible. Because of the stress situation, be sure to pay extra attention that your rate of ascent does not exceed 30 feet/10 metres, per minute.

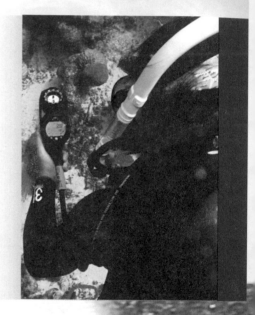

5

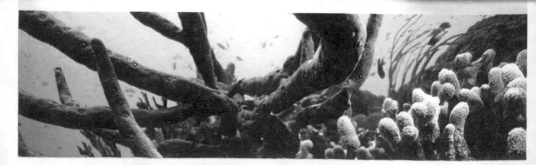

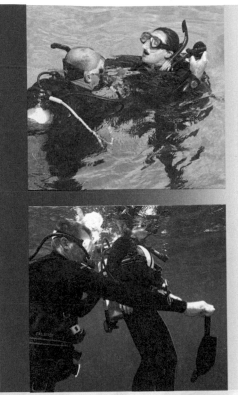

On the Surface, Use Positive Buoyancy

Once you reach the surface, achieve positive buoyancy immediately and make sure your buddy does the same. If your buddy is unable to, then do it for him. If you feel that either you or your buddy needs maximum buoyancy, drop your weight. If your buddy is clinging to you for security, a properly fitted, full-capacity BC jacket should support his or her weight also. This should dispel your fears of being drowned by your buddy, and should make you feel safe to offer physical support instead of pushing your buddy away from you. However, you may have reason to question the flotation ability of your BC if your buddy significantly outweighs you, or if you are wearing an older, smaller BC.

If at any time you feel endangered, push your buddy away, kick him or her with your fins, or descend below the surface out of reach.

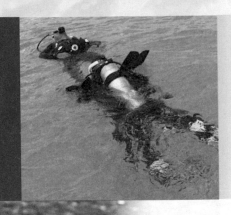

Help Your Buddy with a Simple Tow if Necessary

If your buddy is too tired to swim safely to the shore or boat, help with a simple tow. Whenever performing a tow, pace yourself and swim in a relaxed manner, alternating fin kicks to relieve muscle fatigue.

5

Buddy Rescue

A buddy rescue is required when the victim is out of control. At this point divers cannot think clearly, make decisions, or control their actions. Their instinct is to get out of the water and into open air at all costs. They may become dangerous to you at this point, lacking the ability to respond to you logically, and possibly using you merely as a means to obtain their goal. Panicking victims may knock your air source from your mouth, or may use you as an object to climb on in an attempt to secure their own safety.

Skills Needed for Buddy Rescue

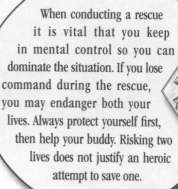

When conducting a rescue it is vital that you keep in mental control so you can dominate the situation. If you lose command during the rescue, you may endanger both your lives. Always protect yourself first, then help your buddy. Risking two lives does not justify an heroic attempt to save one.

The skills needed for a buddy rescue are more complex than buddy assist skills because you are dealing with someone in immediate danger. The rescue can be complicated by excessive stress, injury, a dive malady such as embolism, or the need to search for a lost victim. Since most rescues involve a diver in panic, these skills revolve around saving divers who are incapable of saving themselves.

1. **All buddy assist skills**
2. **Handling a struggling buddy**
   a. Under water
   b. On the surface
3. **Rescue breathing**
4. **Searching for a missing diver**
   a. Lost buddy procedures
   b. Search procedures

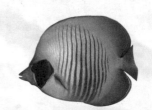

Handling a Struggling Buddy

The worst panic situation occurs under water. Luckily, it is also very rare. But if it ever does happen, visual contact may be the first step in calming the victim down. If you feel you are in danger, remain below the victim; a struggling diver's main objective is to reach the surface, and it is not a good idea to interfere with this objective if the diver is truly out of control.

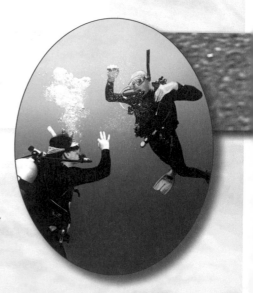

If there is some confusion as to which way is up — which is entirely possible — visual contact and coaxing motions on your part may help, but stay clear of the buddy.

Struggling divers on the surface are also dangerous, but your chances of calming them down increase. Your BC should provide you with enough support, when fully inflated, to help your buddy without putting you in jeopardy.

While assisting a panicking buddy at the surface, always keep your mask on and your second-stage regulator in your mouth so that you can push off from your buddy with your legs and descend below the surface of the water to escape injury. A panicking diver will not follow you if you go back under water.

Rescue Breathing

Every diver should know how to perform rescue breathing (mouth-to-mouth resuscitation) on land, but in the water two quick breaths to ventilate the victim and attempt to restore breathing is adequate.

In the water two quick breaths to ventilate the victim and attempt to restore breathing is adequate.

Rescue breathing in water is not only extremely difficult, it may delay your exit to shore or boat, and it may also force more water into the lungs. It is recommended to get your victim out of the water as soon as possible; help may be nearby or waiting on the boat.

One factor to consider is the distance you are from the boat or shore. If you are a long distance away, you may consider more intensified in-water rescue breathing. However, the overall consideration before beginning rescue breathing is whether the diver has a pulse. Dry suits, hoods, and extremely cold water may make it difficult to determine whether a pulse is present. If no pulse is detected, it is of the upmost importance to get the victim back to shore as quickly as possible. In this situation, rescue breathing should be performed in the water, but should be done in conjunction with CPR once the victim is on the shore or boat.

In-water CPR should not be attempted. It is ideal to get the victim out of the water before a serious and prolonged attempt is made to revive him or her. In-water CPR may also pose the risk of forcing gastric stomach contents into the victim's lungs.[1]

Searching for a Missing Buddy

A lost buddy procedure should always be decided on in the pre-dive phase. Some of the things to consider are how long you should search before surfacing, how long you should wait on the surface, whether you should descend on any bubbles you see, and how long you should wait before getting help. Always be mentally prepared for a search in case you ever get separated from your buddy.

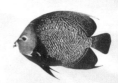

Generally, if you do not spot the diver under water after making two 360 degree visual sweeps of the area, you should surface. Making a lengthy swimming search initially wastes time and may lead to further separation. Once on the surface, if bubbles cannot be seen after a reasonable waiting period, you should assume the diver is in trouble and send for help.

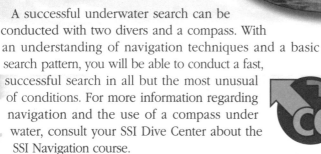

A successful underwater search can be conducted with two divers and a compass. With an understanding of navigation techniques and a basic search pattern, you will be able to conduct a fast, successful search in all but the most unusual of conditions. For more information regarding navigation and the use of a compass under water, consult your SSI Dive Center about the SSI Navigation course.

Search Equipment

Two pieces of equipment — a compass and a buoy — are necessary for conducting a diver search. Additional markers on shore should be used to mark the search area.

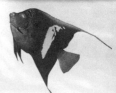

Search Techniques

1. Start by establishing the last-seen point of the missing diver and marking that area on shore by placing markers to designate the search area.

[1]Steven Linton, Damon A. Rust & T. Daniel Gilliam, *Dive Rescue Specialist Training Manual* (Fort Collins: Concept Systems, 1986), p. 9

2. Using a reciprocal compass heading of the course the missing diver was following, begin a systematic search of the last seen area by starting at one end and working to the other end.

3. After each sweep have someone on shore drop a buoy or marker on shore to mark the start of the next sweep.

4. Search sweeps should overlap slightly.

5. Remember to consider the amount of nitrogen accumulated by the searching divers and their available air supply. Then plan the search according to depth and bottom time limitations that may apply.

6. If visibility is good enough to see the bottom, you can utilize the same techniques, but can snorkel on the surface to eliminate excessive bottom time and reduce the risk to searchers.

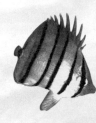

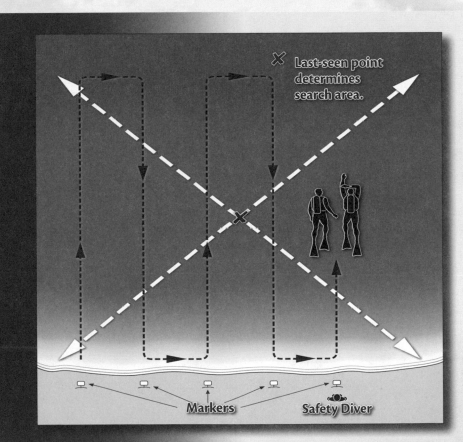

Last-seen point determines search area.

Markers   Safety Diver

Search technique using two divers, a compass, and a safety diver on shore.

Search Pattern Checklist

1. The search team (two divers and one shore person) must agree on the search pattern and the marking system for the area to be searched.

2. The search divers must check all equipment and insure that they both have enough air to execute the search.

3. The shore person should brief the divers on the dive plan and any limitations to depth and bottom time.

4. The search team should formulate a plan for the rescue or recovery of the missing diver when found, and coordinate the notification of professional rescue or medical assistance and transportation to the nearest medical facility.

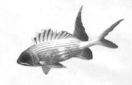

For a more in-depth look at search patterns and techniques, consider enrolling in the SSI Search and Recovery specialty course offered by your SSI Dive Center.

Procedures to Protect Yourself and Perform a Buddy Rescue

When rescuing a buddy there are precautions you can take to protect yourself from danger. First and foremost is remaining calm and in control.

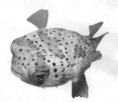

Never attempt a rescue without the full use of your equipment, including mask, fins, snorkel, and some type of flotation such as a BC or wet suit. If you are not able to see, breathe, and float, you will not be able to help your buddy without endangering yourself.

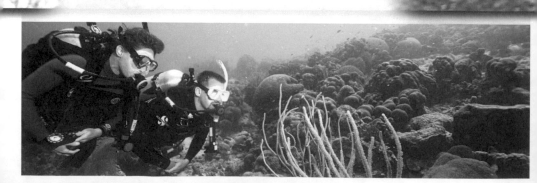

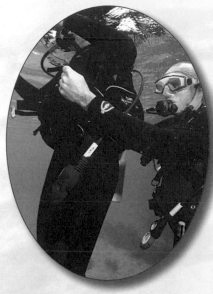

Inflate your buddy's BC and drop his weights, either by keeping his cylinder between you, or by dropping below the surface out of reach.

Performing a Rescue Under Water

1. Approach the victim, stopping at a safe distance to detect the cause of panic.

2. Attempt to calm the victim through eye contact, hand signals, then physical contact.

3. Be prepared at all times to push away from the victim or escape by descending.

4. If you receive no response from your buddy, achieve positive buoyancy for both of you by inflating the victim's BC and dropping the weight if necessary.

5. Proceed to the surface, controlling your buddy's buoyancy as well as possible. If it becomes impossible to control your buddy's buoyancy, let go of him or her and control your own.

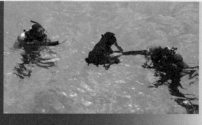

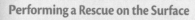

Performing a Rescue on the Surface

1. Use maximum positive buoyancy to protect yourself. Use a surface flotation device if available.

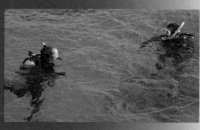

2. Approach the victim slowly, stopping at a reasonable distance to assess the situation.

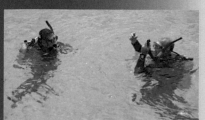

3. Try to get the victim to establish positive buoyancy (if not already done) by instructing him or her to inflate the BC and/or drop the weight belt.

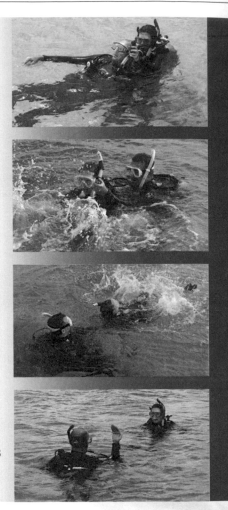

4. Attempt to calm the victim through vocal communication, visual and physical contact. If you receive no response, you must inflate the BC and drop the weight belt for your buddy.

5. If the diver is hysterical, make them positively buoyant by inflating the BC and dropping the weight belt either from behind, by keeping the victim's cylinder between you, or by dropping below the surface out of reach.

6. If the victim remains hysterical, tow him or her from behind, making it impossible for them to reach you, or place a flotation device between you and the victim.

7. When the diver regains control, continue helping them to shore with a tow, or lead the way to safety by swimming ahead and giving verbal instructions for them to follow.

Rescuing an Unconscious Diver

The worst case scenario in diver rescue is finding your buddy unconscious under water. This situation is unlikely, but you still need to be prepared for it.

When rescuing an unconscious diver time is of the essence. No matter how you attempt the rescue, the most important thing to do is get the victim to the surface and begin resuscitation. First aid cannot be administered under water. In this situation, panic on your part could be deadly. You must remain mentally alert and physically capable. You must also remember that any time you feel that you are in danger, you should stop until you feel it is safe to continue.

Skills Needed to Rescue an Unconscious Diver

If you find a diver unconscious under water, assume there is some chance for survival and proceed accordingly. You will not have much time to think once you discover your buddy, so you must be ready to act immediately. First, remember to stay in control and prevent panic in yourself. Listed below are skills you should mentally rehearse in order to be prepared for this situation.

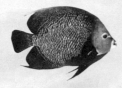

1. All buddy rescue skills including searching for a missing diver

2. Bringing an unconscious diver to the surface

3. Handling an unconscious buddy on the surface

4. Transporting an unconscious buddy to boat or shore

5. Getting an unconscious buddy onto the boat or shore

Bringing an Unconscious Buddy to the Surface

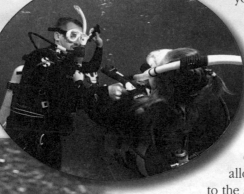

Controlling the ascent with your BC.

When bringing your buddy to the surface, you need to do it as quickly as possible. Use positive buoyancy to get both of you and the victim to the surface. By using buoyancy, you decrease your chance of becoming fatigued. Dragging a victim while ascending can be physically exhausting.

One method is to remove the unconscious diver's weights, then control the ascent with your BC. This allows you to let the victim free-float to the surface if you must let go to control yourself or your rate of ascent.

Handling an Unconscious Buddy on the Surface

When you arrive at the surface, achieve positive buoyancy for both of you. Conserve your energy for your return to the boat or shore. Again, stay in mental control, using deep breathing to relax. Immediately check the victim's ABCs: open the victim's Airway, check for Breathing, and check the Circulation to see if a pulse is present. All of these indicators will help determine how fast you must work and how quickly you'll need to get outside help.

Transporting an Unconscious Buddy to the Shore or Boat

The decision on how long to spend helping your buddy in the water should be based on his/her vital signs.

Practical Notes

If you are wearing gloves, remove them before checking for vital signs, and if you are wearing a dry suit with seals at the wrists, your sense of feeling may not be delicate enough to detect a pulse.

If the victim has no pulse or heartbeat, it is pointless to attempt any in-water resuscitation. You should get the victim out of the water as quickly as possible so you can perform adequate CPR.

As discussed earlier in this book, in-water CPR is inefficient and even dangerous. Immediate care will help sustain the victim but is no substitute for evacuation to an emergency medical facility. Time is of the essence.

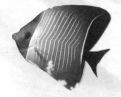

If the victim is not breathing but has a pulse, your decision on your level of care will be based on your distance from the shore or boat. Perform rescue breathing by opening the airway and giving the victim two quick breaths before you begin the trip to the shore or boat. If you have a long way to swim and you were not able to restore breathing, continue to give the victim one breath every five seconds until you reach safety. This procedure will of course be easier with the help of another diver.

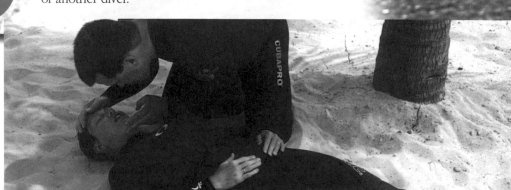

Getting your Buddy onto the Shore or Boat

Before attempting to lift an unconscious diver into a boat or onto shore, remove and ditch the victim's equipment. It is up to your own discretion whether or not to keep your own on. If you must complete the exit alone, your equipment may be a hindrance and add to your fatigue.

The three most common exits will be onto a boat, onto a beach, or over rocks at a shore line.

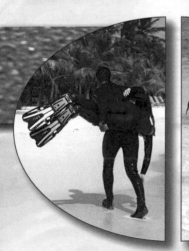

A rope or net is helpful when hoisting an unconscious diver aboard a boat.

Helping your buddy onto a boat can be difficult, especially if it is not equipped with a ladder or platform. A rope or net is helpful when hoisting an unconscious diver aboard a boat with a high freeboard. In this situation the roll up technique works well. By rolling the victim up the side, you avoid having to use brute strength. On a boat whose deck is closer to the water, a simple lifeguard hoist might work. Once you are in the boat, simply lift the victim by the arms until you get his/her stomach over the edge of the boat. There are a variety of ways to get an unconscious diver aboard a boat, and they will vary according to the type of boat and the conditions; it may take some innovative thinking to figure out the best way, given the particular circumstances.

If you are exiting onto a beach, use a tow and allow the surf to carry you in as far as possible. As you enter the surf zone, use your body to block incoming waves so that your buddy does not inhale or swallow water. Once on shore you can use a saddle-back carry

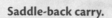

Saddle-back carry.

or Packstrap carry to get the victim up onto the beach.

Getting your buddy onto shore over rocks is a difficult skill, so use extreme caution. Wait until the waves hit a lull before swimming towards the rocks. Grab onto the rocks, bracing yourself for the next set of waves. As soon as there is another break in the waves, climb onto the rocks, rolling or lifting the victim after you. You may need to wait for another lull in the waves before climbing any farther.

Any method of exit will be performed more safely and easily with the help of another person.

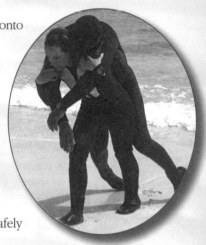

Packstrap carry.

Review of Procedures for
Rescuing an Unconscious Diver

Care should be taken when handling an unconscious diver. Rough handling can complicate unseen injuries. Again, speed is critical, but not as important as your own safety. Below is a step-by-step list of what to do when rescuing an unconscious diver.

1. Locate the victim, using a search pattern if necessary. Use any available help.

2. Remove the victim's weights and return to the surface as quickly as possible. Keep the victim's body vertical, with head tipped back to keep the airway open.

3. Control your ascent. If the combined buoyancy of you and the victim results in too rapid an ascent, you may want to release the victim and regain control, either rejoining the victim or allowing him or her to ascend alone to the surface.

4. Once you reach the surface, achieve positive buoyancy, removing your weight if necessary.

5. Place the victim in a face-up position, remove the mask and regulator, and inflate the BC. This will allow the victim to float and to breathe the open air.

6. Check the ABCs.

   A = *AIRWAY:*
   Be sure there are not obstructions.

   B = *BREATHING:*
   If the victim is not breathing, give 2 quick breaths to open airway.

   C = *CIRCULATION:*
   Check pulse, and if there is no heartbeat, begin CPR as soon as you can get the victim on the shore or boat.

7. If the shore or boat is at a great distance, tow your buddy as quickly as you feel you can without becoming exhausted. Use any assistance available.

8. When on shore or boat, administer immediate care as described in Section 4 — "Accident Management".

Summary

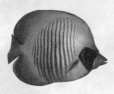

This section is an extremely important source for divers who wish to be safe and self-assured, and who value being vigilant and dependable dive buddies. The skills we have mentioned here should be overlearned, and should be reviewed often. One of the most important areas of stress management in diving is the knowledge of how to act in an emergency.

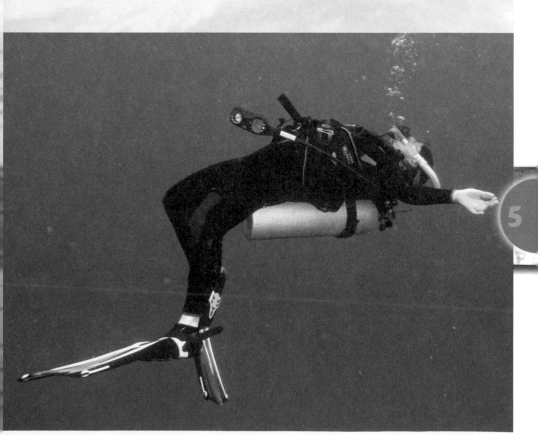

Section 5 Review Questions

1. An out-of-air situation is the most critical and demands immediate attention, but in most cases, "_____ – _____ – _____ – _____" is the best way to regain control and make an intelligent decision.

2. A _____ _____ is used when a _____ is experiencing stress but is still under control.

3. Choose the _____ that is safest and easiest for the environment and situation.

4. The physical and visual _____ provided by this (side-by-side) tow gives your buddy a sense of _____ .

5. The surface float works with a _____ _____ because it keeps you and the victim separated, and allows the victim to rest with their _____ above water so they can relax and get under control.

6. Always remember to take care of yourself first without your safety, both of your _____ could become _____ .

7. If you are unsure about your buddy's _____ _____ , stop out of reach until you can assess the _____ .

8. If you are on the surface, establish _____ _____ first in case your buddy becomes _____ .

9. If at any time you feel _____ , push your buddy away, kick him or her with your fins, or _____ _____ the surface out of reach.

10. A _____ _____ is required when the victim is out of control.

11. _____ _____ in water is not only extremely difficult, it may delay your exit to shore or boat, and it may also force more water into the lungs.

12. Never attempt a rescue without the full use of your equipment, including _____ , _____ , _____ , and some type of _____ such as a BC or wet suit.

13. If you find a diver _____ under water, assume there is some chance for _____ and proceed accordingly.

14. If the victim has no _____ or _____ , it is pointless to attempt any in-water _____ .

15. Any method of _____ will be performed more safely and easily with the help of another person.

5

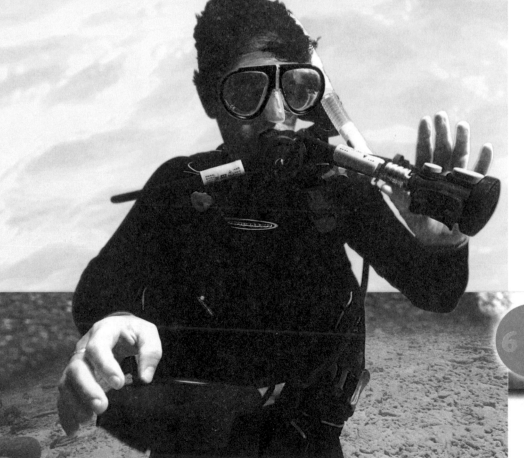

Conditions That Complicate Rescues

Complications During Rescues

Many conditions can complicate self-aid, buddy assists, and rescues. This is, again, why it is important that you have good skills, knowledge, equipment, and experience. Your control will help overcome complications caused by the environment, cold water, or injury. If you lose control when other complications are present, the chances of failure and accident increase.

Section 6 Objectives

After completing this section you will be able to describe conditions that may complicate a rescue, including:

♦ The environment,

♦ Water movement,

♦ Impairments and injuries,

♦ Hypothermia/cold water.

The Environment

Poor environmental conditions, particularly limited visibility and excessively cold water, will make rescues more difficult. Poor visibility will make it harder to locate buddies, and notice difficulties and monitor them. Cold water can impair your mental processes as well as lower your physical dexterity. Motor skills such as inflating a BC can be affected by extreme cold, and can be further complicated by restrictive equipment such as dry suits, hoods and gloves. The agility of the fingers is one of the things most affected by cold.

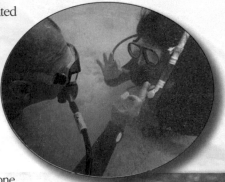

Limited visibility can complicate rescues.

A change in environmental conditions is one reason so many accidents happen in Stage 3, after the dive. The water environment is a powerful force and can change from moment to moment. Poor conditions will even test the strength of healthy, strong divers, and can overwhelm panicked, injured, and fatigued divers.

Water Movement

Water movement such as surf, surge, waves, and currents can also complicate rescues. Fighting against a current or a rough surface can rob you of strength, especially if your diving route has taken you far from your entry point. Communication can be difficult, and rescue skills such as tows and weight ditching become more difficult when water is thrashing at you. Mental control is imperative in such circumstances.

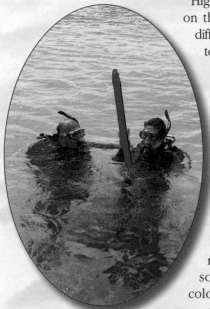

High seas will also limit your ability to see divers on the surface, making rescues of lost divers difficult. There are a few precautions you can take to prevent the possibility of being stranded on the surface in rough seas. The first and easiest precaution to is always have a reserve of air. Many boat operators recommend you surface with 1000 pounds/70 bar of air and locate the boat. You can then take a compass heading and drop below the surface for the return swim. You will not have a very good chance of making a long surface swim back to the boat in rough seas; this is why you need a reserve of air so you can swim under water.

An inflatable surface marker is useful in high seas.

If, however, you do get stranded with no reserve of air, there are still a few precautions so you will be easier to recognize. Brightly colored wet suits and BCs will help make you more noticeable, especially when your BC is fully inflated so you are floating as high above the water as possible. Carry a whistle to call for help. The sound of a whistle will carry farther and longer than the sound of your voice. One last suggestion, and requirement of some operators, is to carry an inflatable surface marker. This marker fits in your BC pocket and stands around 7 feet/2 metres out of the water when fully inflated.

Impaired Movement

Coral, kelp, wrecks, and fishing nets can all impair movement, creating stress and complicating the rescue process. Any time you lack a full range of movement it will be more difficult to help yourself or another person.

Stress and loss of patience can worsen the situation by causing further entanglement. In order to rescue divers who are entangled, you must first calm them so they stop struggling. Once you are both relaxed, you can proceed with the rescue. Entrapment in ice or caves is a serious situation. The only way to safely dive in these situations is through proper training and preventative measures. Once loss of direction or entrapment occurs, there is little hope of rescue.

SSI does not recommend diving in either ice or caves without proper training because of the danger involved.

Injury

Ear drum rupture, cuts, bites, stings and other injuries can cause severe pain and contribute to panic. Buddies may have a difficult time helping themselves or thinking clearly because of their injury. Again, make an effort to calm the victim, assuring him or her that they will be okay and are not in any life-threatening danger, and then help them get safely back to the shore or boat. Once you are on solid ground you can administer proper first aid to the injury and send for help if necessary. Basic first aid for marine bites and stings can be found in your SSI Open Water Diver manual.

Heart Attack

Exhaustion, age, poor physical fitness, cold, improperly fitted equipment, and panic are but a few of the contributors to heart attack when diving. Many of these victims are predisposed to cardiac arrest, and the stresses of diving can actually trigger an attack.

If you or any diver is ever experiencing shortness of breath or chest pain on the surface, the dive should be cancelled and the victim should be helped to the shore or boat immediately for help. Be careful to help the victim back to the exit point so they don't overexert and trigger a heart attack.

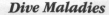

Dive Maladies

Overexpansion injury and decompression sickness are the two most common dive maladies, and like all diving injuries require immediate attention from qualified medical personnel. Good dive buddies should understand the basic symptoms of the most common diving injuries so they can administer first aid and provide details to medical personnel. When an expansion injury or decompression sickness is suspected, the victim should be administered pure oxygen. It is especially important for dive leaders and others who are responsible for divers to have access to and know how to administer 100% oxygen. The symptoms and treatment of diving maladies is covered in Section 4.

Cold Water Near-Drowning

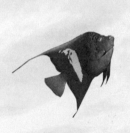

It is now possible for people who have drowned in cold water to be resuscitated after up to one hour of submersion without brain damage. The cold water near-drowning victim is able to stay alive due to a slowing down of blood circulation to tissues, muscles, and non-vital organs, which greatly reduces the body's need for oxygen. The blood is channeled to the essential organs — the heart, lungs and brain. The survival rate is highest in infants and small children, but many adults have also survived without brain damage.

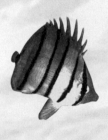

The most widely publicized factor contributing to cold water near-drowning has been a physiological trait of sea mammals, the Mammalian Diving Reflex. However, recent research points to a variety of other factors, the most prominent of which is general hypothermia.[1]

[1]Steven Linton, Damon A. Rust & T. Daniel Gilliam, *Dive Rescue Specialist Training Manual* (Fort Collins: Concept Systems, 1986), p. 6

Remember that if a diver apparently drowns in cold water there may be a chance for survival, and, therefore, you should act as if there is; even if the victim displays classic signs of death such as blue skin, rigidity, and the absence of pulse.

Treatment

Treatment for cold water near-drowning victims is a delicate procedure, best accomplished by trained medical personnel at an emergency medical facility.

1. Open airway and give two quick breaths.
2. Administer CPR.
3. Contact emergency medical personnel.
4. Administer 100% oxygen.
5. Warm the body in the field by applying a pre-warmed blanket around the body, leaving the arms and legs uncovered. Get the victim to room temperature. (Note: Warming is a delicate procedure and should be done by medical personnel only.)

Hypothermia

Hypothermia is generally defined as the condition of having one's body temperature fall below normal. The term is also used to describe the overall effects of severe cold on a victim. This refers to exposure to cold temperature either in the water, topside, or both.[2] Some levels of hypothermia are instant, such as falling overboard into freezing waters, other levels build throughout the day as you are subjected to chilled waters and a long windy boat ride back to shore. The most susceptible areas of your body to heat loss are the head, underarms and groin. This is another reason why it is so important to wear adequate thermal protection when diving, adding a vest and hood for protection. In water below 65°F/18°C, it is highly advised to wear a dry suit. Your SSI Dive Center offers a Dry Suit Specialty course on the proper use of dry suits.

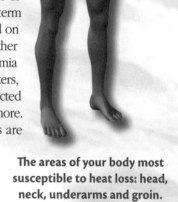

The areas of your body most susceptible to heat loss: head, neck, underarms and groin.

Because the only three ways to heat your body are by fuel intake (food), exercise, or adding layers of insulation (clothing, blankets, etc.), most people wake up in the morning in a slightly hypothermic state. The first symptom of mild hypothermia is shivering,

[2]Steven Linton, Damon A. Rust & T. Daniel Gilliam, *Dive Rescue Specialist Training Manual* (Fort Collins: Concept Systems, 1986), p. 6

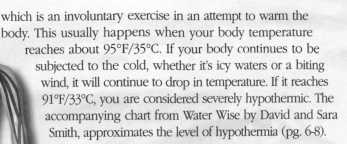

which is an involuntary exercise in an attempt to warm the body. This usually happens when your body temperature reaches about 95°F/35°C. If your body continues to be subjected to the cold, whether it's icy waters or a biting wind, it will continue to drop in temperature. If it reaches 91°F/33°C, you are considered severely hypothermic. The accompanying chart from Water Wise by David and Sara Smith, approximates the level of hypothermia (pg. 6-8).

As the body's metabolism continues to lower its rate, and the blood centres in the brain and heart, the hypothermia victim's pulse will continue to drop. Once the core temperature drops below 86°F/30°C, you may not be able to detect a heartbeat, even though the heart is still beating, because the tissues are poor sound conductors at these temperatures.[3] For this reason, it is best to get the victim out of the water as quickly as possible so you can begin warming and recheck the ABCs.

Treatment

Treatment for hypothermia is much the same as for the cold water near-drowning victim, except the hypothermia victim may be breathing and have a pulse. If this is true, CPR should not be administered.

Do not begin CPR unless you are positive that no pulse is present; performing CPR on a beating heart can cause the rhythm to alter, possibly causing the heart to stop. (Take a one-minute carotid pulse on each side of the throat in very cold patients.)

1. Open airway and give two quick breaths. Rescue breathing will help to internally warm the victim.
2. Begin CPR if no pulse is detected.
3. Warm the victim (as discussed in cold water near-drowning).
4. Handle the victim gently. Do not rub or squeeze the victim in an attempt to increase warmth or circulation.
5. Keep the victim's movement to a minimum.
6. Transport to an emergency medical centre.

[3]Dave and Sarah Smith, *Water Wise* (St. Charles: Smith Aquatic, 1984), p. 125

Levels of Hypothermia
(General approximations — patients may vary)

°F	°C	Physical Response
99.6	37.6	Normal rectal temperature.
96.8	36.0	Increased metabolic rate in attempt to balance heat loss.
95.0	35.0	Shivering maximum at this temperature.
93.2	34.0	Patients usually responsive and normal blood pressure.
91.4	33.0	Severe hypothermia below this temperature.
89.6	32.0	Consciousness clouded, pupils dilated*, most shivering ceases.
87.8	31.0	Blood pressure difficult to obtain.*
86.0	30.0	Progressive loss of consciousness. Increased muscular rigidity.
85.2	29.0	Slow pulse and respiration; cardiac arrhythmia develop.
82.4	28.0	Ventricular fibrillation may develop if heart irritated.
80.6	27.0	Voluntary motion lost along with pupillary light reflex, deep tendon and skin reflexes appear dead.*
78.8	26.0	Victims seldom conscious.
77.0	25.0	Ventricular fibrillation may appear spontaneously.
75.2	24.0	Pulmonary Edema develops.
73.4	23.0	
71.6	22.0	Maximum risk of fibrillation.
69.8	20.0	Heart standstill.
66.2	19.0	
64.4	18.0	Lowest accidental hypothermic patient with recovery.
62.6	17.0	iso — electric eeg
48.2	9.0	Lowest artificially cooled hypothermic patient with recovery.

* Do not misinterpret these responses as signs of death in live but very cold victims.

Levels of Hypothermia. (Reprinted from *Water Wise*)

96.8°F/36.0°C ▶
Increased metabolic
rate in attempt to
balance heat loss.

91.4°F/33.0°C ▶
Severe hypothermia
below this
temperature.

These temperatures are
based on 99.6°F/37.6°C
as normal rectal
temperature.

78.8°F/26.0°C ▶
Victims Seldom Conscious.

64.4°F/18.0°C ▶
Lowest accidental hypothermia
patient with recovery.

Rapid warming of the hypothermic victim can be dangerous, even life threatening. Attempt only to stabilize their body temperature, preventing a further decrease. Do not attempt to increase body temperature. The application of hot packs to the victim could cause severe burning and trauma to the skin. Warming should be attempted only by medical personnel.

Summary

Because of the nature of diving accidents, they often occur under less than ideal conditions. The weather may be severe or the seas high. These conditions are another reason that practice of rescue skills is important in order to be able to perform in an actual situation, and especially under poor conditions.

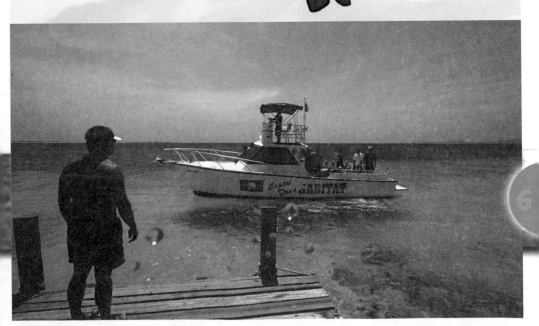

Section 6 Review Questions

1. Your control will help overcome complications caused by the

   _____ , _____ _____ ,

   or _____ .

2. Motor skills such as _____ a BC can

   be affected by extreme cold, and can be further complicated by

   _____ _____ such as dry suits, hoods

   and gloves.

3. _____ _____ such as surf, surge,

   waves, and currents can also complicate rescues.

4. Exhaustion, age, poor physical fitness, cold, improperly fitted

   equipment, and panic are but a few of the contributors to

   _____ _____ when diving.

5. The most widely publicized factor contributing to cold water

   near-drowning has been a physiological trait of sea mammals,

   the _____ _____ _____ .

6. Some levels of _____ are instant, such as

   falling overboard into freezing waters, other levels build throughout

   the day as you are subjected to chilled waters and a long windy boat

   ride back to shore.

7. Once the core temperature drops below 86°F/30°C, you may not

   be able to detect a _____ even though the

   _____ is still beating, because the tissues are

   poor sound conductors at these temperatures.

8. Treatment for _____ is much the

   same as for the _____ _____ _____ –

   _____ victim.

9. Rapid _____ of the hypothermic victim

   can be dangerous, even _____ _____ .

10. _____ should be attempted only by

    medical personnel.

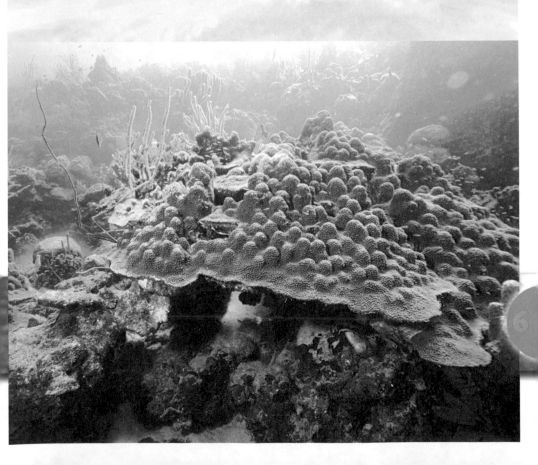

Diver Stress & Rescue: Summary

Diver stress and the resulting panic are the leading causes of diving accidents and fatalities. Many conditions can cause or aggravate stress throughout the three stages of diving: before the dive, during the dive, and after the dive. At any point it should be possible to detect and deal with stress so that the dive can be continued as planned. Early detection, especially in the pre-dive phase, can prevent many problems. If stress is allowed to become extreme, panic and accidents can result.

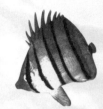

The key to early detection is proper identification. Understanding the physical, mental and physiological causes of stress will help you identify it in yourself and your buddy. Proper identification is essential to solving the stress problem, for without understanding the cause, a proper solution cannot be determined.

Stress can be prevented through precautions such as proper medical attention and physical fitness, proper dive planning, and using quality equipment correctly. If you are truthful with yourself about your physical condition, diving ability, and the relative safety of diving conditions, you will never exceed your diving limits. Inadequate training and unfamiliar conditions can lead to stress, as the diver encounters a situation beyond his or her control.

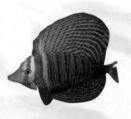

Learn how to detect stress in yourself and practice self-aid skills. Through self-confidence and ability you can stop most stress from progressing. Basic skills such as mask clearing and weight ditching may be enough to avert a diving emergency. The practice of stop-breathe-think-act can help you regain control when stress occurs. Deep breathing can help control the flow of adrenaline through the body and help you regain mental stability.

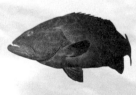

If stress is not stopped early, or other conditions such as fatigue or entanglement interfere, a buddy assist may become necessary. Again, buddies are a safety essential in diving, always ready to lend a hand, provide mental support, and get help if necessary. Diving without a buddy is not recommended.

When stress is allowed to progress beyond the buddy assist level, the chance of panic and accident increase, possibly leading to the need for a buddy rescue. A rescue situation occurs when divers no longer have the ability to control themselves mentally or physically. In a rescue, always protect yourself first; do not put your life in danger when attempting a rescue. You must also remember to stay in control of the situation at all times.

If you yourself feel panic coming on, stop and breathe, then decide on the best course of action.

If a buddy is discovered unconscious under water or on the surface, immediate action is necessary to save his or her life. You must get the victim to the surface and to safety as soon as possible without jeopardizing yourself. Both rescue breathing and CPR are difficult to perform in water, so it is best to get the victim to a hard surface immediately if one of these procedures is necessary.

Safe divers are those who have learned how to prevent, identify, and deal with stress in themselves and others, have good basic skills, stay current in their training, and mentally rehearse emergency skills. They always make a dive plan which includes contingencies for emergencies, and they always stay well within the no-decompression limits of the dive tables.

Safe divers also dive within their limits and do not dive in unfamiliar conditions or without proper training and guidance. An up-to-date, complete, and properly maintained Total Diving System should always be used to help prevent problems, and to help deal with problems if they do occur.

Through all this preparation you can become a stress-free diver and learn how to control stress in any situation.

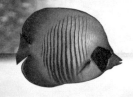

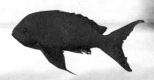

Appendix

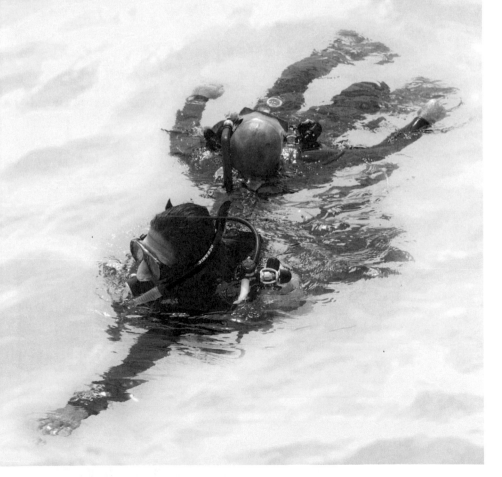

DIVER STRESS & RESCUE
DIVING ACCIDENT
MANAGEMENT FLOW CHART

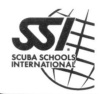

REPRINTED BY PERMISSION FROM THE DIVERS ALERT NETWORK

DIVER WITH SYMPTOMS

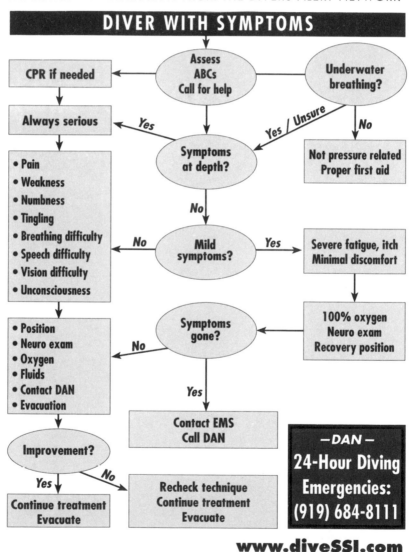

Assess ABCs Call for help

Underwater breathing?

CPR if needed

Always serious

Yes

Yes / Unsure

No

Symptoms at depth?

Not pressure related Proper first aid

- Pain
- Weakness
- Numbness
- Tingling
- Breathing difficulty
- Speech difficulty
- Vision difficulty
- Unconsciousness

No

Mild symptoms?

Yes

Severe fatigue, itch Minimal discomfort

No

100% oxygen Neuro exam Recovery position

- Position
- Neuro exam
- Oxygen
- Fluids
- Contact DAN
- Evacuation

Symptoms gone?

No

Yes

Contact EMS Call DAN

Improvement?

Yes

No

Recheck technique Continue treatment Evacuate

Continue treatment Evacuate

— DAN —
24-Hour Diving Emergencies: (919) 684-8111

www.diveSSI.com

DIVER STRESS & RESCUE
DIVING ACCIDENT
MANAGEMENT FLOW CHART

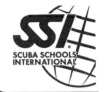

REPRINTED BY PERMISSION FROM THE DIVERS ALERT NETWORK

DIVE PROFILE

Day	Dive #	Depth	Bottom Time	Surface Interval

ACCIDENT INFORMATION

▲ VICTIM'S NAME

▲ ADDRESS

▲ PHONE NUMBER

▲ DATE / TIME

▲ ALLERGIES

▲ MEDICATIONS

▲ IN CASE OF EMERGENCY, CONTACT (Name & Phone Number)

▲ LOCAL MEDICAL FACILITY (Name, Address & Phone Number)

www.diveSSI.com

REVISED 9/95, 1/04, 2/09 • 1561D_0209

Reorder # 2506SR

DIVER STRESS & RESCUE
5-MINUTE **NEURO-EXAM**

NOTE: USING THIS CUE-CARD DOES NOT REPLACE THE NECESSARY TRAINING TO EFFECTIVELY PERFORM A NEUROLOGICAL EXAM.

Perform the following steps and place a check in the box next to any area that has abnormal or questionable results.

☐ **1. ORIENTATION** — Does the diver know his/her own name and age? Does the diver know the present location? Does the diver know what time, day, year it is? Note: Even though a diver appears alert, the answers to these questions may reveal confusion. Do not omit them.

☐ **2. EYES** — Have the diver count the number of fingers you display, using two or three different numbers. Check each eye separately and then together. Have the diver identify a distant object. Tell the diver to hold head still, or you gently hold it still, while placing your other hand about 18 inches/0.5 meters in front of the face. Ask the diver to follow your hand. Now move your hand up and down, then side to side. The diver's eyes should follow your hand and should not jerk to one side and return. Check that the pupils are equal in size.

☐ **3. FACE** — Ask the diver to purse the lips. Look carefully to see that both sides of the face have the same expression. Ask the diver to grit the teeth. Feel the jaw muscles to confirm that they are contracted equally. Instruct the diver to close the eyes while you lightly touch your fingertips across the forehead and face to be sure sensation is present and the same everywhere.

☐ **4. HEARING** — Hearing can be evaluated by holding your hand about 2 feet/0.6 meters from the diver's ear and rubbing your thumb and finger together. Check both ears moving your hand closer until the diver hears it. Check several times and compare with your own hearing. Note: If the surroundings are noisy, the test is difficult to evaluate. Ask bystanders to be quiet and to turn off unneeded machinery.

☐ **5. SWALLOWING REFLEX** — Instruct the diver to swallow while you watch the "Adam's apple" to be sure it moves up and down.

☐ **6. TONGUE** — Instruct the diver to stick out the tongue. It should come out straight in the middle of the mouth without deviating to either side.

☐ **7. MUSCLE STRENGTH** — Instruct the diver to shrug shoulders while you bear down on them to observe for equal muscle strength. Check diver's arms by bringing the elbows up level with the shoulders,

www.diveSSI.com

Reorder # 2506SR

hands level with the arms and touching the chest. Instruct the diver to resist while you pull the arms away, push them back, up and down. The strength should be approximately equal in both arms in each direction. Check leg strength by having the diver lie flat and raise and lower the legs while you resist the movement.

☐ **8. SENSORY PERCEPTION** — Check on both sides by touching lightly as was done on the face. Start at the top of the body and compare sides while moving downwards to cover the entire body. Note: The diver's eyes should be closed during this procedure. The diver should confirm the sensation in each area before you move to another area.

☐ **9. BALANCE & COORDINATION** — Note: Be prepared to protect the diver from injury when performing this test. **1.** First, have the diver walk heel to toe along a straight line while looking straight ahead. **2.** Have her walk both forward and backward for 10 feet or so. Note whether her movements are smooth and if she can maintain her balance without having to look down or hold onto something. **3.** Next, have the diver stand up with feet together and close eyes and hold the arms straight out in front of her with the palms up. The diver should be able to maintain balance if the platform is stable. Your arms should be around, but not touching, the diver. Be prepared to catch the diver who starts to fall. **4.** Check coordination by having the diver move an index finger back and forth rapidly between the diver's nose and your finger held approximately 18 inches/0.5 meters from the diver's face. The diver should be able to do this, even if you move your finger to different positions. **5.** Have the diver lie down and instruct him to slide the heel of one foot down the shin of his other leg, while keeping his eyes closed. The diver should be able to move his foot smoothly along his shin, without jagged, side-to-side movements. **6.** Check these tests on both right and left sides and observe carefully for unusual clumsiness on either side.

IMPORTANT NOTES

• Tests 1, 7, and 9 are the most important and should be given priority if not all tests can be performed. • The diver's condition may prevent the performance of one or more of these tests. Record any omitted test and the reason. If any of the tests are not normal, injury to the central nervous system should be suspected. • The tests should be repeated at 30- to 60-minute intervals while awaiting assistance in order to determine if any change occurs. Report the results to the emergency medical personnel responding to the call. • Good diving safety habits would include practicing this examination on normal divers to become proficient in the test. • Examination of an injured diver's central nervous system soon after an accident may provide valuable information to the physician responsible for treatment. • The On-Site Neuro Exam is easy to learn and can be done by individuals with no medical experience at all.

DAN EMERGENCY NUMBER   919-684-8111

OTHER NATIONAL AGENCY EMERGENCY NUMBER:_____

DOPPLER NO-DECOMPRESSION LIMITS
BASED ON U.S. NAVY DIVE TABLES

SSI®
SCUBA SCHOOLS INTERNATIONAL

TABLE 1 — No-Decompression Limits and Repetitive Group Designation Table For No-Decompression Air Dives

How to Use TABLE 1: *Find the planned depth of your dive in feet or metres at the far left of Table 1. Read to the right until you find the time (minutes) you plan to spend at that depth. Read down to find the Group Designation letter.*

DEPTH feet / metres		Doppler No-Decompression Limits (minutes)											
10	3.0		60	120	210	300							
15	4.5		35	70	110	160	225	350					
20	6.0		25	50	75	100	135	180	240	325			
25	7.5	245	20	35	55	75	100	125	160	195	245		
30	9.0	205	15	30	45	60	75	95	120	145	170	205	
35	10.5	160	5	15	25	40	50	60	80	100	120	140	160
40	12.0	130	5	15	25	30	40	50	70	80	100	110	130
50	15.0	70		10	15	25	30	40	50	60	70		
60	18.0	50		10	15	20	25	30	40	50			
70	21.0	40		5	10	15	20	30	35	40			
80	24.0	30		5	10	15	20	25	30				
90	27.0	25		5	10	12	15	20	25				
100	30.0	20		5	7	10	15	20					
110	33.0	15			5	10	13	15					
120	36.0	10			5	10							
130	39.0	5			5								

GROUP DESIGNATION: A B C D E F G H I J K

How to Use TABLE 2:

Enter with the Group Designation letter from Table 1. Follow the arrow down to the corresponding letter on Table 2. To the left of these letters are windows of time. Read to the left until you find the times between which your surface interval falls. Then read down until you find your New Group Designation letter. Dives following surface intervals of more than 12 hours are not repetitive dives.

TABLE 2 — Residual Nitrogen Timetable For Repetitive Air Dives

REPETITIVE GROUP AT THE BEGINNING OF THE SURFACE INTERVAL

A	B	C	D	E	F	G	H	I	J	K
0:10 / 12:00*										
3:21 / 12:00*	0:10 / 3:20									
4:50 / 12:00*	1:40 / 4:49	0:10 / 1:39								
5:49 / 12:00*	2:39 / 5:48	1:10 / 2:38	0:10 / 1:09							
6:35 / 12:00*	3:25 / 6:34	1:58 / 3:24	0:55 / 1:57	0:10 / 0:54						
7:06 / 12:00*	3:58 / 7:05	2:29 / 3:57	1:30 / 2:28	0:46 / 1:29	0:10 / 0:45					
7:36 / 12:00*	4:26 / 7:35	2:59 / 4:25	2:00 / 2:58	1:16 / 1:59	0:41 / 1:15	0:10 / 0:40				
8:00 / 12:00*	4:50 / 7:59	3:21 / 4:49	2:24 / 3:20	1:42 / 2:23	1:07 / 1:41	0:37 / 1:06	0:10 / 0:36			
8:22 / 12:00*	5:13 / 8:21	3:44 / 5:12	2:45 / 3:43	2:03 / 2:44	1:30 / 2:02	1:00 / 1:29	0:34 / 0:59	0:10 / 0:33		
8:51 / 12:00*	5:41 / 8:50	4:03 / 5:40	3:05 / 4:02	2:21 / 3:04	1:48 / 2:20	1:20 / 1:47	0:55 / 1:19	0:32 / 0:54	0:10 / 0:31	
8:59 / 12:00*	5:49 / 8:58	4:20 / 5:48	3:22 / 4:19	2:39 / 3:21	2:04 / 2:38	1:36 / 2:03	1:12 / 1:35	0:50 / 1:11	0:29 / 0:49	0:10 / 0:28

NEW GROUP DESIGNATION: A B C D E F G H I J K

REPETITIVE DIVE DEPTH ▼ RESIDUAL NITROGEN TIMES DISPLAYED ON REVERSE ▼

© 1990 CONCEPT SYSTEMS, INC.   Reorder #2190   1120D_0402_SSI_DiveTbl Wall A

DOPPLER NO-DECOMPRESSION LIMITS BASED ON U.S. NAVY DIVE TABLES

TABLE 3 — Residual Nitrogen Times (Minutes)

— CONTINUED FROM REVERSE SIDE —

■ = ADJUSTED NO-DECOMPRESSION TIME LIMITS   N/L = NO LIMIT

REPETITIVE DIVE DEPTH feet	metres	A	B	C	D	E	F	G	H	I	J	K
10	3	39 / N/L	88 / N/L	159 / N/L	279 / N/L							
20	6	18 / N/L	39 / N/L	62 / N/L	88 / N/L	120 / N/L	159 / N/L	208 / N/L	279 / N/L	399 / N/L		
30	9	12 / 193	25 / 180	39 / 166	54 / 151	70 / 135	88 / 117	109 / 96	132 / 73	159 / 46	190 / 15	
40	12	7 / 123	17 / 113	25 / 105	37 / 93	49 / 81	61 / 69	73 / 57	87 / 43	101 / 29	116 / 14	
50	15	6 / 64	13 / 57	21 / 49	29 / 41	38 / 32	47 / 23	56 / 14	66 / 4			
60	18	5 / 45	11 / 39	17 / 33	24 / 26	30 / 20	36 / 14	44 / 6				
70	21	4 / 36	9 / 31	15 / 25	20 / 20	26 / 14	31 / 9	37 / 3				
80	24	4 / 26	8 / 22	13 / 17	18 / 12	23 / 7	28 / 2					
90	27	3 / 22	7 / 18	11 / 14	16 / 9	20 / 5	24 / 1					
100	30	3 / 17	7 / 13	10 / 10	14 / 6	18 / 2						
110	33	3 / 12	6 / 9	10 / 5	13 / 2							
120	36	3 / 7	6 / 4	9 / 1								
130	39	3 / 2										

HOW TO USE TABLE 3: Enter with the New Group Designation letter from Table 2. Next, find the planned depth of your repetitive dive in feet or metres at the far left of Table 3. The box that intersects the Repetitive Dive Depth and the New Group Designation will have two numbers. The top number indicates the Residual Nitrogen Time. The bottom number indicates the maximum Adjusted No-Decompression Time Limit for the next dive.

WARNING: The U.S. Navy Dive Tables were designed to Navy specifications for use by Navy Divers. When used by recreational divers, the tables should be used conservatively. Even when used correctly with proper safety procedures, *decompression sickness may still occur.*

SAFETY STOP PROCEDURE: It is recommended that you make a 3- to 5-minute safety stop at 15 feet (5 metres) on all dives over 30 feet (9 metres).

OMITTED DECOMPRESSION PROCEDURE: Should you exceed the Doppler No-Decompression Time Limits by less than 5 minutes on any dive, it is recommended that you ascend normally to 15 feet (5 metres) and stop for at least 10 minutes or longer if your air supply allows. Should you exceed the Doppler No-Decompression Time Limits by more than 5 minutes but less than 10 minutes on any dive, it is recommended that you stop at 15 feet (5 metres) for at least 20 minutes or longer if your air supply allows.

Refrain from any further scuba diving activities for at least 24 hours.

Works Cited

Bachrach, Arthur, Glen Egstrom. *Stress and Performance in Diving*.
San Pedro: Best, 1987.

Benson, Herbert. *The Relaxation Response*.
New York: William Morrow, 1975.

Faelton, Sharon, David Diamond. *Take Control of Your Life*.
Emmaus: Rodale, 1988.

Goliszek, Andrew. *Breaking the Stress Habit*.
Winston-Salem: Carolina P, 1987.

Griffiths, Tom. *Sport Scuba Diving in Depth*.
Princeton: Princeton Brook, 1985.

Jeppessen Sanderson. *Open Water Sport Diver Manual*.
Vol. 1. Englewood: Jeppessen, 1987.

Linton, Steven J., Damon A. Rust, and T. Daniel Gilliam.
Dive Rescue Specialist Training Manual.
Fort Collins: Concept Systems, 1986.

Mebane, G. Yancey M.D., editor. *DAN Dive & Travel Medical Gude*.
Durham: Divers Alert Network, 1995.

Mebane, G. Yancey M.D., Arthur P. Dick M.D. DAN
Underwater Diving Accident Manual. Durham: Duke UP, 1985.

Merkel, Jim. "More Education, Data Center Director Says."
Underwater USA. Nov 1987: 4.

Pia, Frank. "Observations of Drowning of Non-Swimmers."
The Journal of Physical Education. July/Aug. 1978.

Smith, Dave and Sarah. *Water Wise*.
St. Charles: Smith Aquatic, 1984.

Teather, Corporal R.G. *The Underwater Investigator*.
Fort Collins: Concept Systems, 1983.

University of Rhode Island. U.S.
Underwater Diving Fatality Statistics, 1986-87. URI.

Witkin-Lanoil, Georgia. *The Male Stress Syndrome*.
New York: New Market, 1986.

Wood, John T. *What Are You Afraid Of?*
Englewood Cliffs: Prentice-Hall, 1976.

Wood, Mike. *Dive Control Specialist Handbook*.
Fort Collins: Concept Systems, 1986.

Work, Kathy R.N. *Med Dive Textbook*.
Fort Collins: Dive Rescue Inc./International, 1990.

Index

Student Answer Sheet Directions

- Transfer your Section Review answers to the following six Answer Sheet pages.

- Remember to write your name and the date on each page.

- Sign each page after you have reviewed each incorrect answer with your instructor.

- Your instructor will collect these pages during your Diver Stress & Rescue course.

STUDENT ANSWER SHEET

STUDENT NAME   PART #   DATE

Reviewed and Corrected by Student and Instructor:

STUDENT SIGNATURE   INSTRUCTOR SIGNATURE

1. _____
2. _____
3. _____
4. _____
5. _____
6. _____
7. _____
8. _____
9. _____
10. _____
11. _____
12. _____
13. _____
14. _____
15. _____
16. _____
17. _____
18. _____
19. _____
20. _____

STUDENT ANSWER SHEET

STUDENT NAME   PART #   DATE

Reviewed and Corrected by Student and Instructor:

STUDENT SIGNATURE   INSTRUCTOR SIGNATURE

1. _____
2. _____
3. _____
4. _____
5. _____
6. _____
7. _____
8. _____
9. _____
10. _____
11. _____
12. _____
13. _____
14. _____
15. _____
16. _____
17. _____
18. _____
19. _____
20. _____

STUDENT ANSWER SHEET

STUDENT NAME PART # DATE

Reviewed and Corrected by Student and Instructor:

STUDENT SIGNATURE INSTRUCTOR SIGNATURE

1. _____
2. _____
3. _____
4. _____
5. _____
6. _____
7. _____
8. _____
9. _____
10. _____
11. _____
12. _____
13. _____
14. _____
15. _____
16. _____
17. _____
18. _____
19. _____
20. _____

STUDENT ANSWER SHEET

STUDENT NAME _____ PART # _____ DATE _____

Reviewed and Corrected by Student and Instructor:

STUDENT SIGNATURE _____ INSTRUCTOR SIGNATURE _____

1. _____
2. _____
3. _____
4. _____
5. _____
6. _____
7. _____
8. _____
9. _____
10. _____
11. _____
12. _____
13. _____
14. _____
15. _____
16. _____
17. _____
18. _____
19. _____
20. _____

STUDENT ANSWER SHEET

STUDENT NAME   PART #   DATE

Reviewed and Corrected by Student and Instructor:

STUDENT SIGNATURE   INSTRUCTOR SIGNATURE

1. _____
2. _____
3. _____
4. _____
5. _____
6. _____
7. _____
8. _____
9. _____
10. _____
11. _____
12. _____
13. _____
14. _____
15. _____
16. _____
17. _____
18. _____
19. _____
20. _____

STUDENT ANSWER SHEET

STUDENT NAME   PART #   DATE

Reviewed and Corrected by Student and Instructor:

STUDENT SIGNATURE   INSTRUCTOR SIGNATURE

1. _____
2. _____
3. _____
4. _____
5. _____
6. _____
7. _____
8. _____
9. _____
10. _____
11. _____
12. _____
13. _____
14. _____
15. _____
16. _____
17. _____
18. _____
19. _____
20. _____